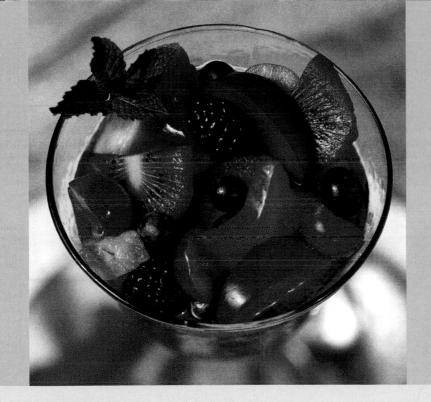

DR. RICHTER'S

produce for
healthy living
guide

Try-Foods International, Inc.
207 Semoran Commerce Place
Apopka, Florida 32703
Printed in the United States of America
To reorder call 1-800-421-8871

are you living healthy?

ONE OF THE BEST WAYS TO FEEL HEALTHY IS TO EAT THE foods that help put your body and mind in sync. We all want to enjoy what we eat, and feel satisfied and "full" at the end of a meal. Yet, complicated, multi-ingredient recipes are usually too time-consuming to prepare. There are hundreds of quick fix diets, each having its authority figure behind it. The lack of long-term results makes it tempting to go back to what you

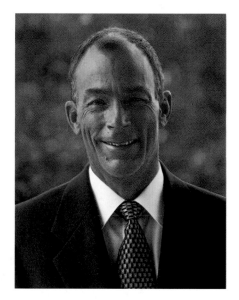

always have done...grab a bite here and there, never having a feeling of control. What about those extra pounds?

So how do you break out of the fast-food, take-out, "just nuke it" mode and put nutritious meals on the table that your family will like, and that you have time to prepare? How do you wade through all the confusing health food information that's currently available?

In my first book, *Dr. Richter's Fresh Produce Guide*, I introduced you to the amazing variety of fresh, healthy produce available at America's grocers. Many of you discovered new foods, or new ways to prepare them. And your families liked them!

HENRY RICHTER,
M.D.

Read on as I take some of the mystery out of eating well, for the reader who is trying to prevent heart disease, the parent who wants her children to learn healthy habits, or the senior citizen concerned about cancer and other diseases of the aged. Produce is nature's ammunition.

Throughout this book, you'll see how to use fruit and vegetables to liven up every meal and snack. There are many produce selections to choose from. Fruit and vegetables add a gold mine of taste to all you serve. So go to your grocer, fill the cart with a variety of fresh produce and set your table for a healthy tomorrow. Check with your doctor prior to dramatically altering your diet. Eat well!

H J Richter

Henry Richter, M.D.

contents

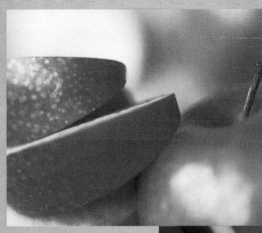

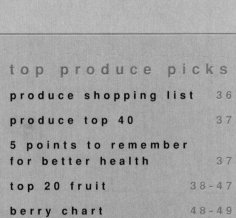
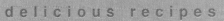

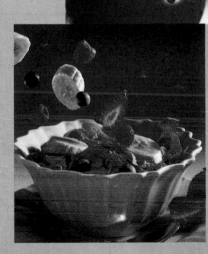

healthy living for real life

YOU HAVE A FAST-PACED LIFE, filled with the demands of work, family, friends and other obligations. How do you fit healthy eating into your day?

It's easy to eat well once you know the secret. Simply stock up on produce during your weekly shopping trip.

When you start the week with a bountiful supply of nature's goodness in your kitchen, it's amazing how easily healthy eating fits into your life!

In this book, you will learn how to increase the total amount of food you can eat without gaining weight. It's quick and easy to substitute sweet, juicy fruit and tasty, satisfying vegetables for higher density, less satisfying junk or fast foods.

Dr. Richter's Healthy Living Produce Guide provides a wealth of easy-to-understand information about fruit, vegetables and herbs that you can start using right away. Dr. Richter also addresses the most commonly asked questions about the connection between produce, disease prevention and good health.

Finally, to tempt your appetite, the book features a recipe collection of wonderful dishes, categorized by meal occasion. From a hearty breakfast to a festive holiday dessert, you will be surprised (and happy!) to see how fruit and vegetables add delicious flavor and appetizing texture to your meals.

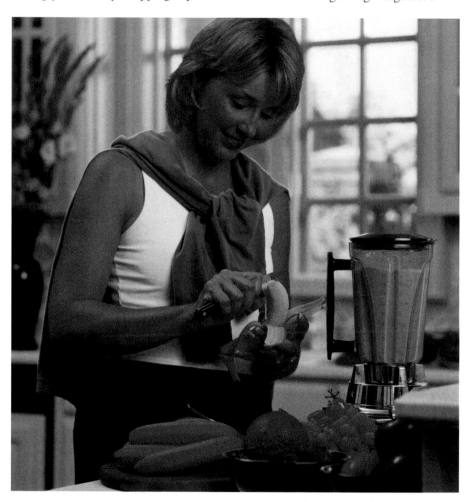

are you getting enough?

How many servings of fresh fruit and vegetables did you and your family eat yesterday? If you're like many Americans, you can double that number and still barely meet the recommended minimums. The Produce for Better Health® Foundation, in coordination with the National Cancer Institute, recommends at least five, and preferably nine, servings of fruit and vegetables a day. Of every five U.S. adults, only one meets that goal, while one skips vegetables completely.

incorporating fruit & vegetables
into your daily diet

FRUIT AND VEGETABLES...THEY'RE EASY TO FIX, delicious to eat and they can help reduce your risk of cancer and heart disease. For optimum health, everyone should eat a diet HIGH in produce and LOW in fat, saturated fat, cholesterol and sodium. The Produce for Better Health® Foundation, in coordination with the National Cancer Institute, coined the phrase "5 A Day—for Better Health!" to help consumers remember this vital fact: Eating five servings of fruit or vegetables daily is a matter of good well-being.

WHAT IS A PRODUCE SERVING?

...smaller than you think. Eating five servings of fruit and vegetables every day is easy when you pick produce at each meal. 1...2...3...4...5! Wake up with the goodness of fruit, then count along throughout the day. By day's end you'll easily reach the goal of at least five fruit or vegetables.

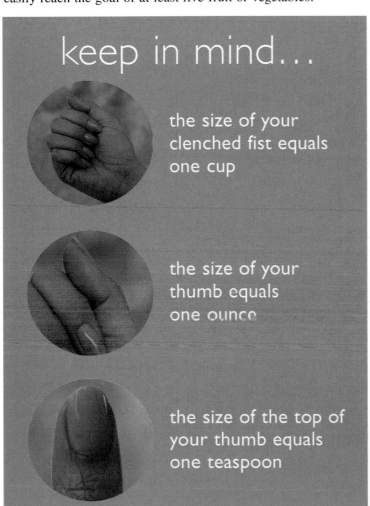

keep in mind...

the size of your clenched fist equals one cup

the size of your thumb equals one ounce

the size of the top of your thumb equals one teaspoon

IN GENERAL, THE USDA SPECIFIES ONE SERVING AS:

1 medium-size piece of fruit or vegetable such as 1 orange or carrot

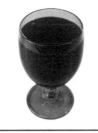 3⁄4 cup (6 oz.) of 100% fruit or vegetable juice

1⁄2 cup cooked or canned fruit or vegetables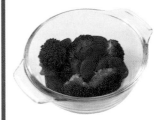

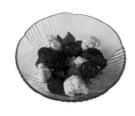 1 cup raw vegetables or leafy greens

1⁄4 cup dried fruit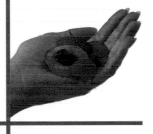

ONE SERVING AT-A-GLANCE

Apple	1 medium	Cherries, fresh	12 large
Apricots, fresh	3 medium	Grapefruit	1⁄2 medium
Artichoke	1⁄2 medium	Raisins	1⁄4 cup
Banana	1 medium	Tomato sauce	1⁄2 cup

grab it & go   simple produce tips

We're all busier than ever these days. Added stress makes it even more important to eat well. The nutrients you receive from fresh produce help keep you energized! Fuel up and remember to count to at least five each day! Here are some easy hints to keep you counting all day long.

FAST FRUIT

Add a handful of fresh berries or slice a banana on your cereal

Take a banana along for the ride

Top waffles with fresh fruit or blend your own fruit purée

Squeeze fresh lemon, lime or orange juice into drinking water

VEG OUT

Pile lettuce and tomatoes on sandwiches

For a shortcut salad, use bagged greens...open the bag and pour out the goodness

Top burgers with mushrooms and onions

Chop fresh vegetables into rice mixes

Send the kids off to school with bagged carrot and celery sticks

TASTIER CHOICES

Go for a portobello burger over the fast-food sandwich

Reach for 100% fruit or vegetable juice instead of a carbonated beverage

Bag the potato chips. Slice cucumbers and dip into a low-fat vegetable dressing

Instead of bread, use a baked potato as the foundation and add your favorite topper

SWEET OPTIONS

Top low-fat ice cream and sorbets with fresh fruit, avoiding sugary syrups

Don't scoop ice cream...scoop a kiwi

Spoon fresh berries into yogurt for a fruitful blast

Satisfy a sweet tooth by dunking strawberries and pineapple chunks into fat-free chocolate dip

FROZEN DELIGHTS

Don't have fresh? Stock frozen fruit to blend for smoothies

Freeze a bunch of seedless grapes for a tantalizing snack

Make ice cubes out of 100% fruit juice

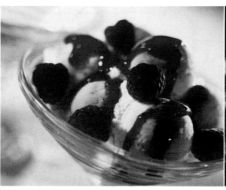
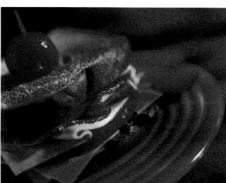
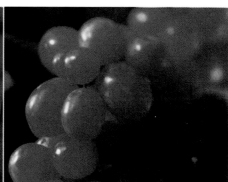

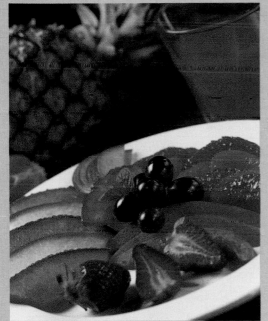

change one meal
at a time

TAKE A LOOK AT WHAT YOU'RE
CURRENTLY EATING. BEGIN EATING
MORE PRODUCE. DR. RICHTER'S
TOP TEN PICKS (SEE PAGE 20) ARE
A GOOD PLACE TO START. CHANGE
A MEAL AT A TIME. FOR INSTANCE,
FOCUS ON A FRUITFUL BEGINNING,
CONSUMING A SERVING OR TWO
FOR BREAKFAST. NEXT WEEK, ADD
A HEALTHY LUNCH AND SO FORTH.
LOOKING AT THE SUGGESTED MENUS
FEATURED ON PAGES 8-13, WHAT
MEAL PARTS ARE EASY FOR YOU TO
CHANGE, STARTING TOMORROW?

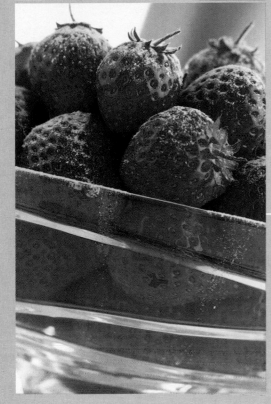

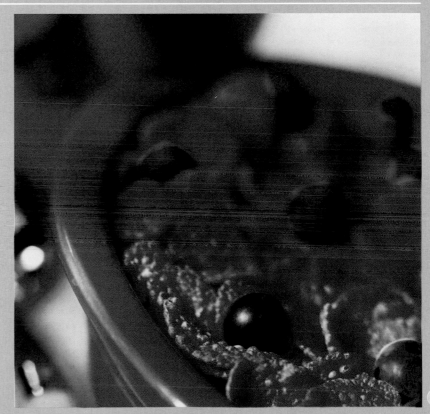

the choice is yours...

YOU MAY BE SURPRISED TO LEARN JUST HOW much of your daily calorie and fat allowance a seemingly innocent breakfast-on-the-go consumes. That little something to get you going in the morning will leave you feeling sluggish before noon. Start your day by eating smart, and not only will you be well on your way to getting your 5 A Day but you'll have energy that lasts.

breakfast

large banana-nut muffin
= 620 calories, 31 g fat

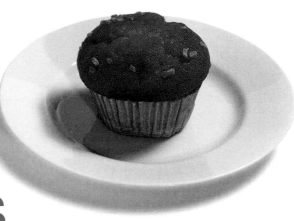

VS

2 bowls shredded
wheat and bran cereal
with skim milk
and bananas

= 620 calories, 3 g fat

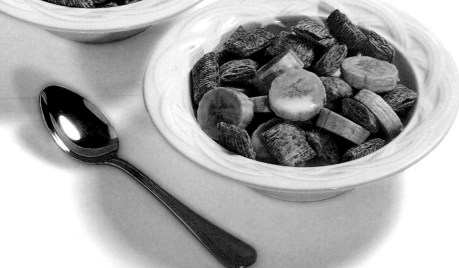

sausage, egg and cheese on

croissant breakfast sandwich

= **530** calories, **41** g fat

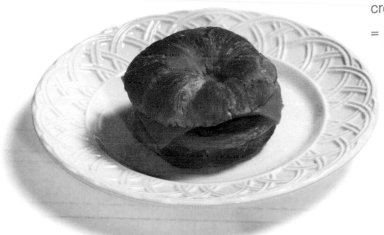

VS

2 eggs with

fresh veggies,

2 slices whole grain toast with jam

and orange juice

= **530** calories, **12** g fat

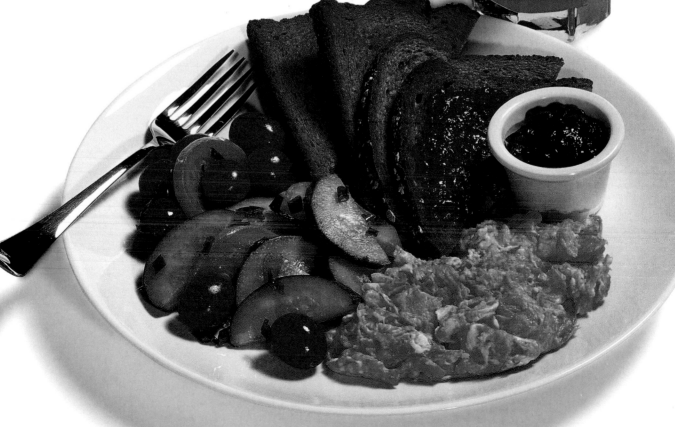

the choice is yours...

YOU MAY BE SURPRISED TO SEE HOW SOME POPULAR lunch choices can sabotage a healthy eating plan. On the other hand, quick and easy-to-make options such as pasta with veggies or a lean meat and vegetable sandwich pack your midday meal with good nutrition.

lunch

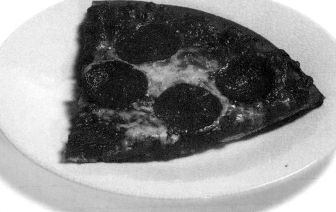

1 slice pizza with pepperoni
= **644** calories, **32** g fat

VS

bowl of pasta with
tomato sauce,
fresh zucchini,
turkey pepperoni,
sprinkle of Parmesan
and toasted roll

= **644** calories, **6** g fat

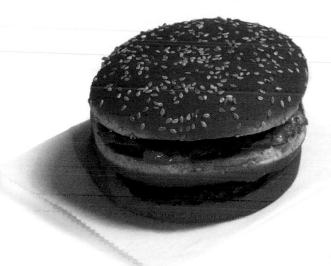

double cheeseburger
= 560 calories, 31 g fat

VS

turkey sandwich with mustard
topped with veggies,
on oatmeal bread,
with fruit salad,
low-fat potato salad
and sparkling water with lime

= 560 calories, 7 g fat

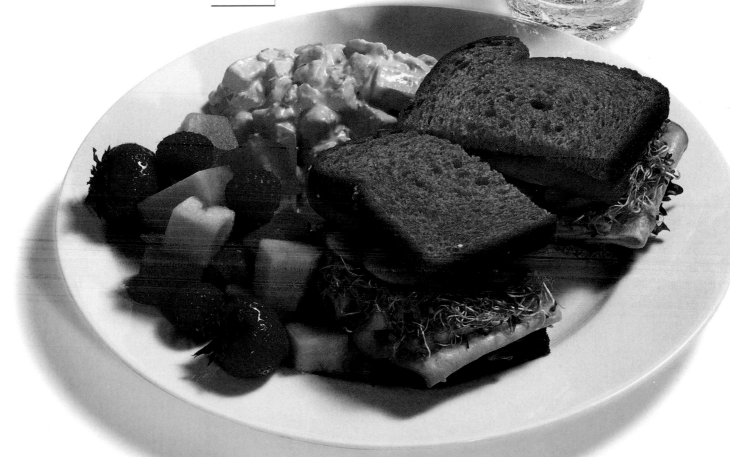

the choice is yours...

YOU MAY BE SURPRISED TO SEE HOW SOME OF the same dinner ingredients can have very different nutritional values when prepared in different ways. It's not necessary to cut favorite foods like potatoes and cheese from your menu, just choose and use them wisely.

dinner

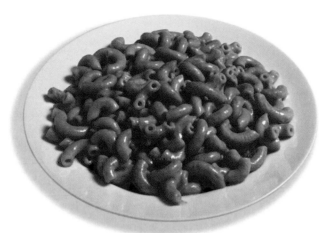

macaroni and cheese casserole
= 772 calories, 36 g fat

VS

vegetable lasagna,
big green salad,
fat-free Italian dressing,
Italian roll and
glass of red wine

= 466 calories,
16 g fat

fried chicken breast, leg and thigh,
macaroni and cheese
and creamed spinach

= 855 calories, 48 g fat

VS

barbecue grilled chicken breast,
green salad,
corn on the cob,
baked potato and
unsweetened iced tea

= 494 calories, 6 g fat

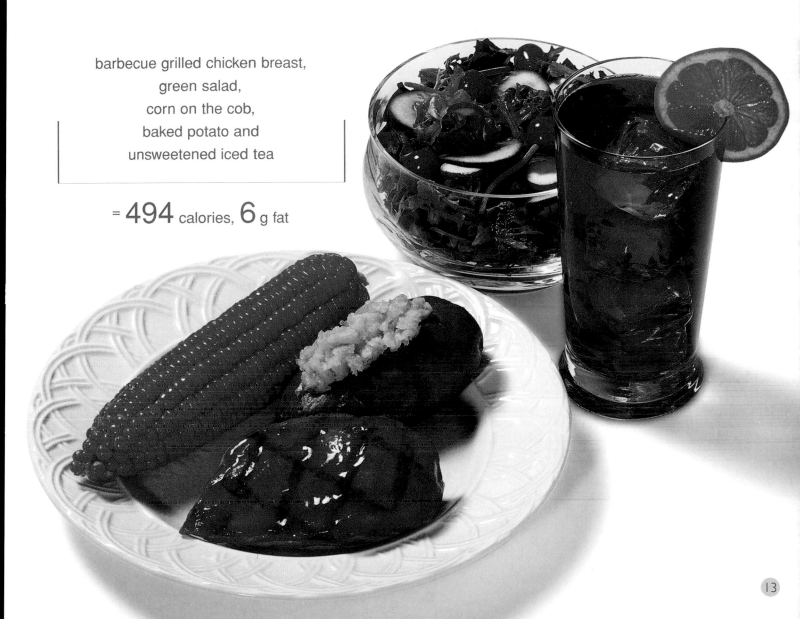

the choice is yours...

SNACKS ARE GREAT TO GIVE YOU A LITTLE energy boost and satisfy cravings. Here you'll see that you can enjoy something crunchy or satisfy your sweet tooth while still eating healthy.

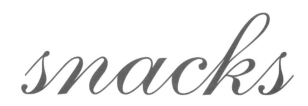

snacks

crudité platter (celery, broccoli florets, bell peppers, baby carrots, zucchini, cherry tomatoes) and hummus dip

= 480 calories, 4 g fat

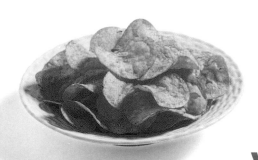

3 oz. potato chips
= 480 calories, 30 g fat

VS

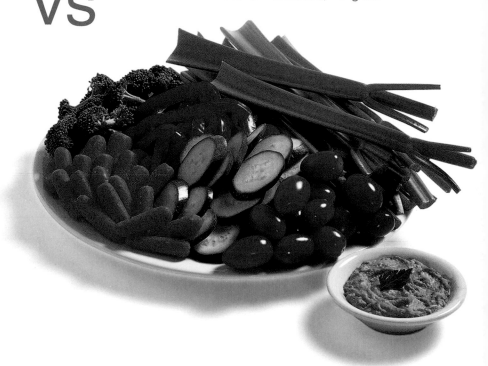

1 chocolate truffle
= 220 calories, 13 g fat

VS

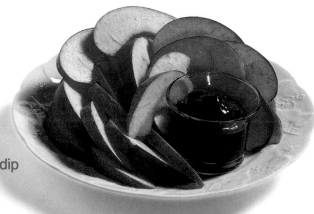

apples and fat-free chocolate dip
= 220 calories, 1 g fat

the choice is yours...

HERE'S PROOF THAT DESSERT CAN BE LUSCIOUS and still be light. Plus it's one more chance to reach your 5 A Day goal.

dessert

1 cup premium chocolate ice cream
= **540** calories, **36** g fat

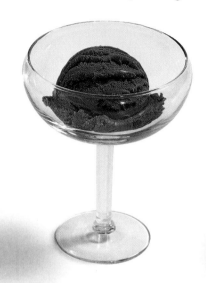

VS

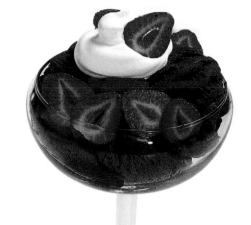

4 cups low-fat chocolate frozen yogurt with fresh strawberries and light whipped topping
= **540** calories, **8** g fat

small slice of blueberry pie
= **360** calories, **15** g fat

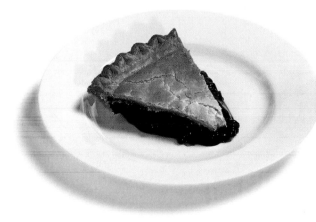

VS

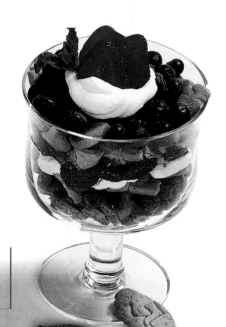

large parfait with blueberries, strawberry slices, light whipped topping and animal crackers
= **360** calories, **9** g fat

long-term weight loss

HIGH-PROTEIN = LOW NUTRITION

While protein is an essential source of nutrients, today's fad of high-protein, low-carbohydrate weight loss diets is not only ineffective over the long-term, but potentially harmful. Why?

• These diets tend to be high in fat with risky unknown effects on body metabolism.

• High-protein diets eliminate carbohydrates, a food group essential for the minerals, vitamins, antioxidants, phytochemicals, fiber and trace elements our bodies require. Most of our carbohydrates are found in fruit, vegetables and grains.

• Food supplements and vitamin pills cannot replace the healing and preventive qualities found in fruit and vegetables, many of which aren't featured on high protein, low-carb diets.

Read the hype surrounding high-protein diet fads with caution. Remember, nature designed fruit and vegetables for a reason. We are supposed to eat a balanced diet including all the essential food groups.

OUR BODIES PREFER SLOW AND STEADY WEIGHT REGULATION

Research has shown that up-and-down weight loss and gain is unhealthy and can make further weight changes more difficult.

Body weight is a function of three things: body type, calorie consumption and energy intake/expense. Genetically, people are either "big boned" (endomorph), medium-sized (mesomorph) or "small-boned" (ectomorph). Bigger bones require more body tissues to support them while smaller bones require less.

Calculating calorie consumption is not rocket science. Carbohydrates and proteins have 4 calories per gram, and fat jumps up to 9 calories per gram. "Calorie-dense" food has more calories per bite than other foods. Because fat adds texture, smoothness and taste, many of these foods have become

American favorites. But the math doesn't lie. A pound of weight, gained or lost, equals 3600 calories. About four double cheeseburgers equal 3600 calories, and 45 apples are also 3600 calories.

That being said, if we eat more calories than we burn, weight gain is inevitable. As a nation, Americans do not burn many calories, opting for sedentary lifestyles. More alarmingly, the average American child spends more hours in front of the TV than at play, or even in school. Doctors report a sharp increase in obesity and diabetes among children.

Any food plan where you eat fewer calories should work if it becomes a habit, and if it is done slowly enough for the body to adapt. But for most people, the body simply does not adapt without some form of increased activity. In fact, some bodies interpret fewer calories as "starvation mode" and metabolisms slow to conserve energy. Add some vigorous movement and suddenly the body is a dramatically more efficient machine. It uses the calories you eat, rather than storing them.

busting diet myths

THERE ARE MANY MYTHS ABOUT FOOD PLANS. HERE'S THE REALITY.

MYTH #1: SKIP A MEAL TO MAKE UP FOR OVEREATING.	**REALITY:** Use total food per week when planning your regimen. Balance that business dinner or social outing with several lighter meals rather simply skipping the next meal (which can lead to snacking on high-fat food to fight hunger).
MYTH #2: NEVER EAT AT NIGHT.	**REALITY:** A 200-calorie snack does not magically grow into 250 calories at bedtime. The body balances food intake and storage over days, not hours.
MYTH #3: THERE'S NO POINT IN WORKING OUT IF YOU CAN'T DO 20 MINUTES OF AEROBIC EXERCISE THREE OR FOUR DAYS PER WEEK.	**REALITY:** ANY exercise, any activity counts. Park at the supermarket parking lot's far end. Walk into the bank or post office instead of using the drive-throughs. And remember that the brain uses more energy while reading, working at a hobby or in conversation than when watching a video.

exercise your options

WHILE EATING WELL IS KEY TO any beneficial food plan, reaching or maintaining good health also requires some amount of exercise. Working physical activity into your life should be undertaken a bit at a time until you can work your way into a routine of steady, moderate exercise. First of all, you won't get burned out too quickly if you start more slowly. Secondly, you're less likely to injure yourself once your muscles and joints are prepared to handle more intense exercise.

The key to a successful exercise program is to find something you like to do! Did you take walks in the woods as a child? Did you love to ride your bike? Go outside and rediscover the freedom of those activities. Or try something that looks like fun, such as in-line skating, ice skating or horseback riding. When you find the activity that's right for you, you'll look forward to exercise.

Finally, if you get bored with exercise, try cross-training. Walk one day, do a yoga video the next and watch TV on your stationary bike on the third. Cross-training has one big benefit— a combination of activities tones *all* of your muscles.

Of course, exercise and participating in sports aren't the only ways to burn calories. Some other examples include:

• Park at the end of the parking lot and walk the distance

CALORIES BURNED IN 15 MINUTES (150 LB. PERSON)	
Aerobics 107	Playing with kids . . 71
Biking (leisurely) . . 143	Running in place . . 143
Bowling 53	Running up stairs 268
Dancing 80	Shopping 41
Fishing 71	Showering 71
Frisbee 53	Stairmaster 107
Gardening 89	Swimming 143
Golf 80	Walking (leisurely) . . 35
Hiking 89	Walking (briskly) . . 80
House cleaning . . . 44	Yoga 71
Jogging 125	

• Hide your TV remote
• Take the stairs instead of the elevator
• Make an evening walk your new family tradition

a healthy mind

PRODUCE HELPS YOU KEEP fit and feel great. A healthy mind is also important. Start at your own pace and with small servings of produce. Your body will need to adjust and get used to the fiber intake. Stay positive and continue to educate yourself on the benefits of eating a variety of fruit and vegetables. Count your produce servings, but don't be crazed about it! Relax and results will happen.

Achieving your 5 A Day goal is easy when you incorporate multi-produce meals into your routine.

• Opt for more green salads.
• Choose vegetable-laden soups.
• Combine your favorite fruits to make an appealing fruit salad.
• Put a variety of vegetables such as zucchini, onions and eggplant on the grill at your next barbecue.

• Add apples, raisins, citrus and other fruit to green salads.

With the U.S. Department of Health and Human Resources, the U.S. Department of Agriculture, the National Cancer Institute and the National Academy of Sciences all recommending that everyone eat a low-fat, high-fiber, produce-rich diet, you have every reason to adopt an attitude that will lead to a healthier, more energetic you!

Fiber Favorites Adding fiber to your diet is extremely beneficial and very easy to do when you choose from the following:

Fruit:	apples, apricots, citrus fruit, grapes, nectarines, peaches, pears, pineapples, plums, prunes, raisins
Vegetables:	broccoli, carrots, corn, peas, potatoes with skins, romaine lettuce, spinach
Legumes and Seeds:	dried beans, peanuts, sunflower and pumpkin seeds

disease prevention

WONDER FOODS

The age-old dictum "eat your vegetables" is as important today as ever. Most fresh fruit and vegetables have little or no fat, cholesterol or sodium. They're also rich in fiber and packed with nutrients. What's more, they only have a few calories (one medium orange supplies only 70 calories!).

By eating fresh fruit and vegetables, you can satisfy your daily need for several vitamins, including vitamin C, folic acid and beta carotene (the building block for vitamin A). Fruit and vegetables also supply generous

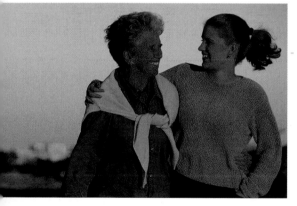

amounts of calcium, iron, magnesium and many of the other vitamins that are essential for good health.

These nutrients help maintain and repair your body's tissues, provide structure for bones and teeth and function in the millions of metabolic processes that keep you healthy, active and energetic. Some studies indicate that people whose diets include lots of fresh fruit and vegetables have significantly lower disease rates.

great news—more is better!

THE BEST ADVICE WHEN IT COMES TO FRUIT AND VEGETABLES IS A FOUR-LETTER WORD—MORE. REPLACING HIGHER-FAT ITEMS WITH MORE FRUIT AND VEGETABLES IS AN EASY, DELICIOUS WAY TO CUT CALORIES AND FAT WITHOUT FEELING DEPRIVED. COMBINED WITH A HEALTHFUL LIFESTYLE, A DIET BASED ON MORE FRUIT AND VEGETABLES IS BENEFICIAL TO GOOD HEALTH.

THE CANCER CONNECTION

The National Cancer Institute estimates that more than one-third of all cancer deaths are related to diet, and could be prevented if people ate more wholesome foods including fruit and vegetables. Most fruit and vegetables contain powerful antioxidants that scientists believe help neutralize free radicals (harmful molecules that hinder the cells' ability to fight cancer).

THE HEART DISEASE LINK

For more than 30 years, the American Heart Association has recommended that people cut back on fat and increase their consumption of carbohydrate and fiber-rich fruit, vegetables, legumes and whole grains in order to lower the risk of developing heart disease. These nutrient-rich foods may help lower blood cholesterol levels, prevent the fatty accumulation in blood vessel walls that leads to heart disease and possibly protect heart tissue from damage.

THE BABY VITAMIN

Pregnant women who eat at least one to two servings each day of folic acid-rich fruit and vegetables may decrease the chances of having a baby with a neural-tube defect, which affects development of the baby's nervous system.

BEYOND VITAMINS & MINERALS

Fruit and vegetables contain thousands of compounds, called phytonutrients or plant nutrients, that may decrease the risk of cancer and stimulate the body's natural immunity to disease.

THE IMPORTANCE OF VITAMINS

Vitamins are powerful substances. A deficiency can cause anemia, bone retardation, blindness, dermatitis, mental illness, overall fatigue or atrophy of tissue. A diet of vitamin-rich foods can help prevent chronic diseases and fight infection. Vital to overall well-being, it may also prevent heart disease, cancer and birth defects.

vitamins & minerals—the natural facts

vitamins & minerals for well-being	chief body functions	other facts	significant produce sources	adult RDA
VITAMIN A & BETA-CAROTENE	Aids in vision, hair, skin, bone, teeth and tissue health	Also aids immune system	Apricots, broccoli, cantaloupe, carrots, mangoes, pumpkin, spinach, squash, Swiss chard, sweet potatoes	900mcg/day
VITAMIN B	Metabolizes amino acids and fatty acids, assists in red blood cell formation	May ease PMS and may help reduce symptoms of stress	Beans, collard greens, escarole, kale, leaf lettuce, nuts, peas, spinach, Swiss chard	2mcg/day
B12 COMPLEX	New cell synthesis, maintains nerve cells, helps to break down fatty and amino acids	Aids nerve metabolism and supports sensation and balance	Animal meats and dairy products. No significant produce source	2mcg/day
FOLATE	Important in new cell formation	Must be consumed daily as it can't be stored	Asparagus, avocados, broccoli, seeds, spinach, beans; garbanzo, green, navy, pinto	200mcg/day, 400mcg/day pregnant woman, heart disease patients
VITAMIN C	May strengthen blood vessels, form scar tissue, support bone growth, strengthen resistance to infection and help in the absorption of iron	May protect against cataracts	Bell peppers, broccoli, Brussels sprouts, cantaloupe, cherries, citrus, jalapeño peppers, lettuce, kiwi, mangoes, papayas, potatoes, spinach, strawberries, tomatoes	60 mg/day, 100mg/day smokers
VITAMIN E	Stabilizes cells, acts as antioxidant	When found in produce may be more useful to the body than when taken in supplement form	Asparagus, avocados, blackberries, corn, kale, kiwi, mangoes, nuts, spinach, Swiss chard, sweet potatoes	10mg/day
VITAMIN K	Helps blood to clot	Deficiency may result in hemorrhaging, jaundice, faulty bile production or diarrhea	Brussels sprouts, cabbage, escarole, kale, Swiss chard, spinach, turnip greens	80mcg/day men 150mcg/day women 215mcg/day pregnant
CALCIUM	Maintains strong bones and teeth, regulates heartbeat assists with blood clotting	Osteoporosis can be caused by insufficient calcium intake as a youngster	Almonds, broccoli, escarole, fortified soy milk, kale, peanuts, spinach, tofu, turnip greens	1,000mg/day 1,200mg/day menopausal woman
MAGNESIUM	Nerve and muscle function	Aids the body's store of potassium, especially important for those on diuretics	Dried beans, green vegetables, nuts, seeds	350mg/day men 280mg/day women
POTASSIUM	Nerve function, heart rhythm	Abundant daily intake (along with calcium and magnesium) may help to regulate blood pressure	Apples, broccoli, citrus, pears, potatoes, tomatoes	2,000mg/day

Dr. Richter's top produce picks for disease prevention

THOSE WHO CONSUME DIETS RICH IN FRUIT AND VEGETABLES MAY PREVENT CERTAIN TYPES OF CANCERS.

Brightly colored fruit and vegetables are packed with antioxidants…blueberries, sweet potatoes and tomatoes all come packed with overflowing goodness. Recent studies show ellagic acid, found in berries, may prevent some cancers. Raspberries and strawberries are a great dessert, supplying fiber for a healthy digestive tract. Forget the battle of the colas— orange or grapefruit juice is all you need to get going.

TOP FRUIT PICKS

fruit	APPLE	BANANA	BERRY	CANTALOUPE	CITRUS	GRAPES (RED)	KIWIFRUIT	MANGO	STONEFRUIT	WATERMELON
phytonutrient/ antioxidant	pectin, flavonoids	pectin, potassium, B6	pectin, Vitamin C, ellagic acid	Vitamin C, potassium, beta carotene	pectin, potassium, limonene	potassium, resveratrol	Vitamin C, magnesium, Vitamin E	potassium, Vitamin C, beta carotene	pectin, carotenes	Vitamin C, fiber, lycopene
possible benefit	heart, cholesterol	heart, cholesterol	cholesterol, cancer	heart, stroke, vision	heart, blood vessels	heart, stroke	blood pressure, heart	heart, blood vessels, vision	cholesterol, vision	prostate, blood pressure

TOP VEGETABLE PICKS

vegetable	ASPARAGUS	BELL PEPPER	BROCCOLI	CABBAGE*	CARROT	GREEN BEANS	SPINACH**	SWEET POTATO	TOMATO	YELLOW ONION
phytonutrient/ antioxidant	folate, potassium, fiber	Vitamin C, lutein	Vitamin C, Vitamin A, flavonoids	Vitamin C, folate, fiber	Vitamin A, beta carotene	fiber	folate, iron, lutein	Vitamin C, potassium, beta carotene	Vitamin C, lycopene	fiber, quercitin
possible benefit	blood vessels, blood pressure	blood vessels	stroke, vision, breast health	breast health, blood vessels	vision, blood vessels	cholesterol	vision, blood vessels	blood pressure, blood vessels	prostate, blood vessels	blood vessels

*AND BRUSSELS SPROUTS

**KALE, SWISS CHARD & COLLARD GREENS ARE GREAT RUNNERS-UPS

the rest of the store

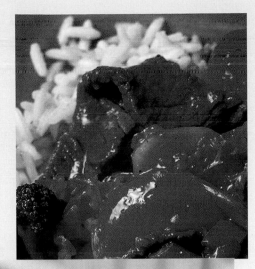

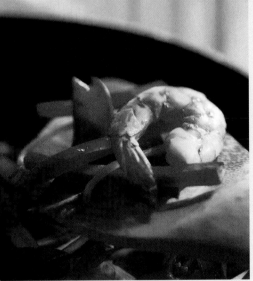

SHOP THE PERIMETER FOR A WEALTH OF GOODNESS

GREAT SOURCES OF nutrition are also found outside of the produce department.

MEAT is an excellent source of protein and essential minerals that are difficult to obtain elsewhere. For instance, red meats are a super source of dietary iron. Currently, approximately three quarters of all American women are deficient in their intake of iron and zinc. The form of iron that is most readily available for your body to digest is heme iron, which is found in meat, poultry and fish. Choose lean meats and avoid the skin. A skinless chicken breast is your best bet for nutrition. Keep meat servings to three ounces, or about the size of your palm.

SEAFOOD is a healthy choice. For instance, wild salmon, albacore tuna, mackerel, Atlantic halibut, shark, rainbow trout and herring contain omega-3 fatty acids. Research has shown that consumption of two servings a week of these types of fish, as part of an overall healthy diet, may reduce your risk of heart disease and some cancers and relieve immune and inflammatory conditions. Omega-3's are believed to increase energy levels and affect fat metabolism. The daily protein recommendation is two to three servings.

BREAD AND GRAINS, including cereal, rice and pasta, contribute complex carbohydrates, riboflavin, niacin, iron, protein, magnesium and fiber. Look for whole grains and enriched breads for maximum nutrient density. The daily grain recommendation is six to 11 servings.

It's okay to occasionally consume butter, salt, salad dressings, mayonnaise or sweets, as long as they're eaten in moderation. However, these foods add little if any nutrient value. Try seasoning with fresh herbs and flavored vinegars instead.

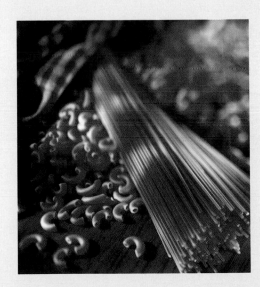

pre-pregnancy eating

WOMEN PLANNING TO BE pregnant may find it easier to find good nutrition advice these days. In fact, "more is more" would be a good motto: more vegetables, fruit, whole grains and limited fat. Each of the major food groups has nutrients for you and your baby, so include a variety of food in your shopping cart.

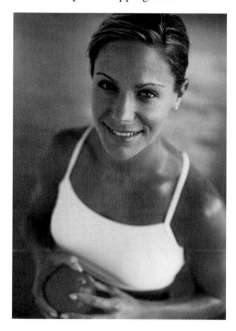

KEEP IT SIMPLE

Fad diets are untested during pregnancy. Ask your doctor about which supplement is best for you. Avoid mega-dose vitamins that may damage your baby.

Good nutrition for a healthy baby starts before you are pregnant. Most prospective mothers can plan for pregnancy to a great degree. Start some strength training exercise

before pregnancy so your back muscles are better tuned to the rigors of the extra weight you will carry. Being in better shape overall will help, too. Weight-bearing exercise such as walking or jogging will put calcium in your bones. Above all, stop smoking and sharply limit your alcohol intake. Both of these habits interfere with the absorption of nutrients you and the baby will need.

IMPORTANT NUTRIENTS

Take advantage of all sources of folate and B vitamins. Folate is vitally important to the very young fetus. Women who typically limit their intake of fortified grains and milk may be folate-deficient in early pregnancy, when the baby needs it most.

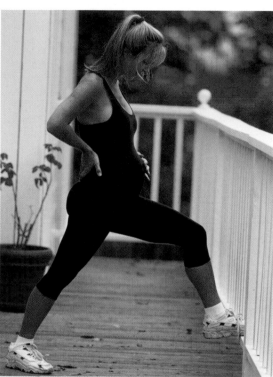

pregnant. Many women who take iron and calcium supplements have problems with constipation and hemorrhoids. Include adequate iron-containing foods like spinach in your diet. Vitamin C will increase iron absorption, a great reason to increase

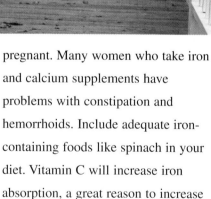

Calcium and iron are two nutrients that require long-term planning.

Calcium and iron are two nutrients that also require long-term planning. Emphasizing foods with these two minerals before pregnancy may decrease the amount of supplementation needed while

the intake of foods with vitamin C at all times.

Calcium is needed for strong bones for the baby. In fact, the placenta will pull calcium from the mother's skeleton if there is not enough available for the

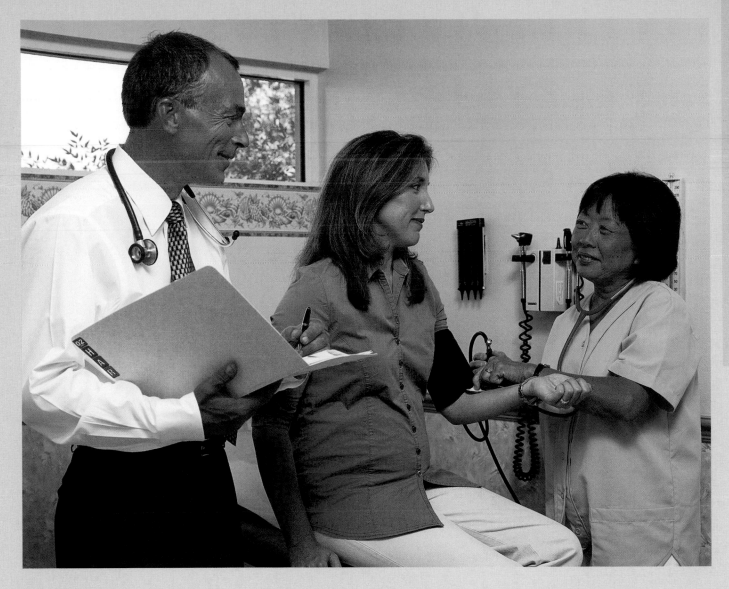

baby. In some cases, this may even cause osteoporosis in the mother.

Studies show possible links to calcium intake during pregnancy possibly benefitting against hypertension.

While pregnant, you should eat a healthy diet. Fruit and vegetables contain the vitamins, minerals, fiber and plant compounds to which our bodies have adapted over thousands of years. The simple sugars in fruit provide pick-up energy during the day. The green leaf vegetables and cruciferous vegetables provide iron and calcium.

The bulk of energy needs should come from several servings of whole grains daily. Most women easily digest starches in these foods. Fats, especially saturated fats, should be limited as

always. Insulin resistance and diabetes are a risk when pregnant, and excess fat and total calories put pregnant women at extra risk of this complication.

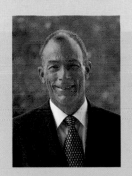

DR. RICHTER SAYS

Eating asparagus, avocado, beans, broccoll, Brussels sprouts, cabbage, carrots, green beans, kale, peas and spinach to boost your folic acid intake may prevent neural-tube defects. Avoid excessive vitamin A intake.

the well-fed child

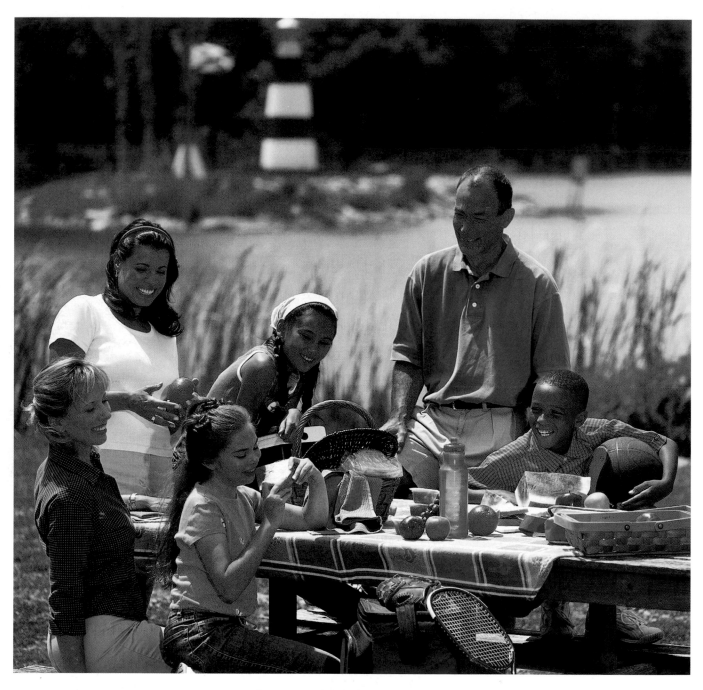

WELL-FED DOES NOT MEAN OVER-FED

We love our children, but when it comes to eating, love may indeed be a matter of "less is more."

There is an epidemic of obesity and subsequent diabetes in American children, which parallels the patterns caused by overeating we see in ourselves, their parents. Vegetarians who consume fat through nuts, seeds or dairy products may have the same weight issues, but far less often than in families eating a more typical American diet. Encourage your child to stop eating when he is full. It is okay to leave food on the plate.

Follow the age/weight tables at your doctor's office, and heed your doctor's advice on overall caloric intake for your child. This is serious business.

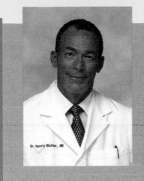

DR. RICHTER SAYS

Eating bananas, a good source of potassium, may provide enhanced muscle and nerve function.

Overeating and under-exercising will affect your child for decades.

HEALTHY CHOICES FOR CHILDREN

A serving size increases by age. For a toddler, a serving of fruit or vegetables is about three tablespoons. This increases to 1/3 cup for the 7-year-old, and to a 1/2-cup adult portion for the teenager. For all children, five or more daily servings of fruit and vegetables are recommended. Nutrients supplied to your child through the various food groups include:

- Meat — protein, iron and B vitamins
- Dairy products — protein, calcium and B vitamins
- Whole or fortified grains — iron, carbohydrates and B vitamins
- Fruit and vegetables — carbohydrates, fiber and vitamins A and C

Feeding your child seems complex because children are naturally fussy. To anxious parents, they may seem to reject food for long periods. Children are learning to handle food on their own. They watch their sibling's, and may at times develop an older sibling's fussiness and taste in food.

Textures, the appreciation of sweetness, tart or sour and the overall "green" taste of vegetables are all new. "Picky" eaters may well be the norm, as most children reject some food groups, with vegetables leading the list.

Help your children grow to like new foods. Do not overfeed at snack time to ensure that your child is hungry at the normal mealtime. Try new foods at the beginning of the meal, when

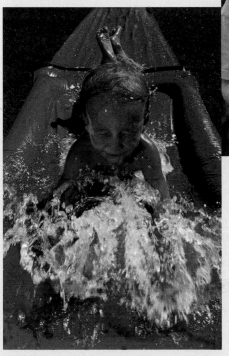

your child is hungriest. Show you enjoy the vegetables you are introducing to your child. And keep trying. As the child grows, he may forget a dislike for a food.

DO CHILDREN NEED SUPPLEMENTS?

Iron, vitamin A, vitamin C and B12 are the most common deficiencies in young children, ages one to three. In vegetarian families, calcium, zinc and riboflavin are additions to the list. School-age girls who diet, and children allowed carbonated beverages are also at risk of calcium deficiency.

Parents often question when they should use supplements. Children drinking non-fluoridated water should receive supplemental fluoride.

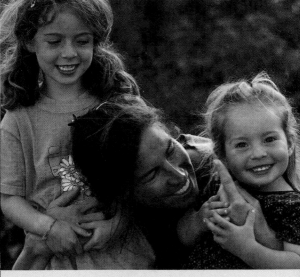

Concerning other nutrients, watch your child's intake of foods over several months. If your child consistently seems to reject the food containing the nutrients discussed above, or eats negligible quantities of them, then supplementation of iron, calcium, or vitamins A, C or the B vitamins may be in order. Always inform your doctor when you are considering a nutrient supplement, so steps may be taken to correct any underlying medical problems.

diabetes awareness plan

ARE YOU ON THE VERGE OF DIABETES?

Diabetes is an epidemic in America. Its twin is obesity, brought on by access to a remote for just about anything, high-fat processed foods for the home and super-sized fast food and restaurant meals. Together, diabetes and obesity are major health issues.

Diabetes attacks your blood vessels, especially the smallest ones, such as in your toes, eyes and kidneys. Diabetes also causes arteriosclerosis, or hardening of the arteries, risking heart disease and strokes. The end result can be blindness, kidney failure and dialysis, and painful, or even amputated feet. Diabetics are two times more likely to have heart attacks, and diabetes compounds the effect of high blood pressure and elevated cholesterol.

Obesity and diabetes go hand in hand. The more fat cells swell with fat, the more they resist the ability of insulin to direct glucose, or sugar, to the muscles that use it to function. The sugar literally "bounces off" the muscle cells, and stays in the bloodstream, where the cascade of damage begins. Doctors call this "insulin resistance," and feel this may be the cause of most diabetes. Depending on your family propensity to insulin resistance, only 5-10 pounds of extra weight in those "love handles" may tip you toward diabetes.

GET ON THE RIGHT TRACK

To reverse the trend to diabetes, plan a more physical lifestyle. Even small amounts of activity help, such as a family walk before dinner, which will also help your children learn healthy habits! Physical activity helps the body burn energy and calories faster. The combination of reduced calorie intake and increased exercise is the best recipe for stalling the onset of or treating diabetes.

Obesity and diabetes go hand in hand.

Remember, losing weight is a goal for your whole life, no matter at what age you start. Favor a slow, habit-forming weight loss of two to four pounds per month. That is 250-500 fewer calories per day, or for example, one less hot dog and a brisk half-hour walk.

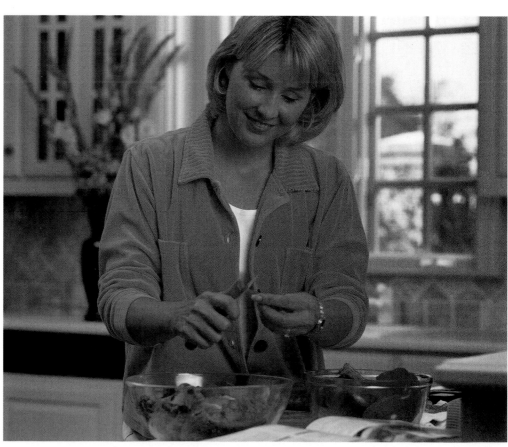

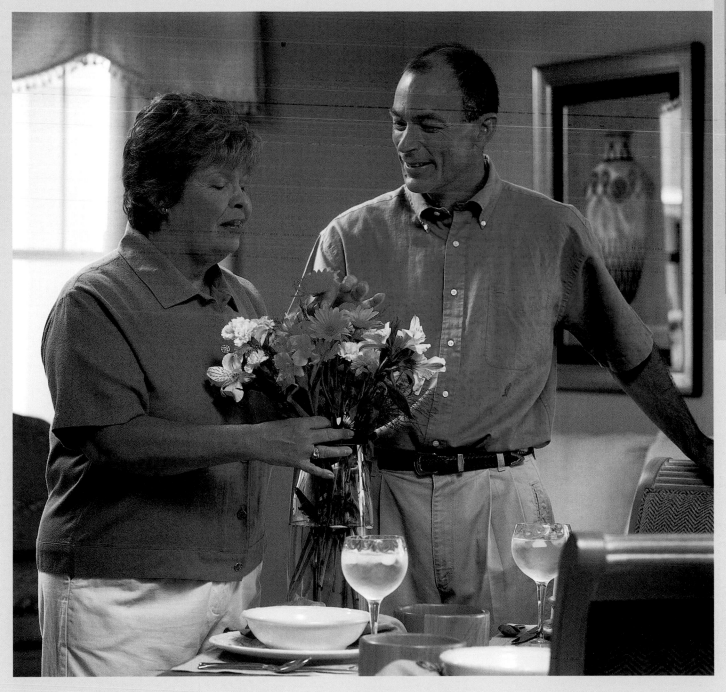

Opt for fresh fruit as dessert. Fruit, vegetables and fortified grains, full of complex carbohydrates, are also loaded with the fiber, antioxidants, phytonutrients, minerals and vitamins we need. Fiber tends to lower absorption of sugars and cholesterol from the intestine.

Reducing the risks of premature illness is multifaceted. But eating properly and exercising will always be a treatment for diabetes, and may lower the dose of medication required, even if it cannot be dispensed with entirely.

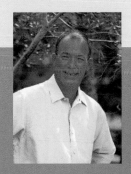

DR. RICHTER SAYS

Eating bananas, garlic, Jerusalem artichokes (sunchokes) and tomatoes may play a beneficial role in the fight against diabetes.

27

heart healthy hints

A LIFETIME JOURNEY — EATING WELL FOR YOUR HEART

HEART DISEASE BEGINS IN CHILDHOOD. Not at 40, when you may have your first cholesterol measurement, and not at 60, when the first heart attack may occur. As a result of the typical American diet, cholesterol streaks — the first sign of cardiovascular disease — are found in children under 10 years old.

PREVENTING THE FIRST HEART ATTACK

Lowering cholesterol and treating high blood pressure are key in helping to ensure that the first heart attack never takes place. Why? Reducing LDL cholesterol by 50 points, say from 180 to 130, may halve the personal risk of a heart attack or stroke.

Prevention is something that you can practice, every day. Since the earliest signs of blood vessel

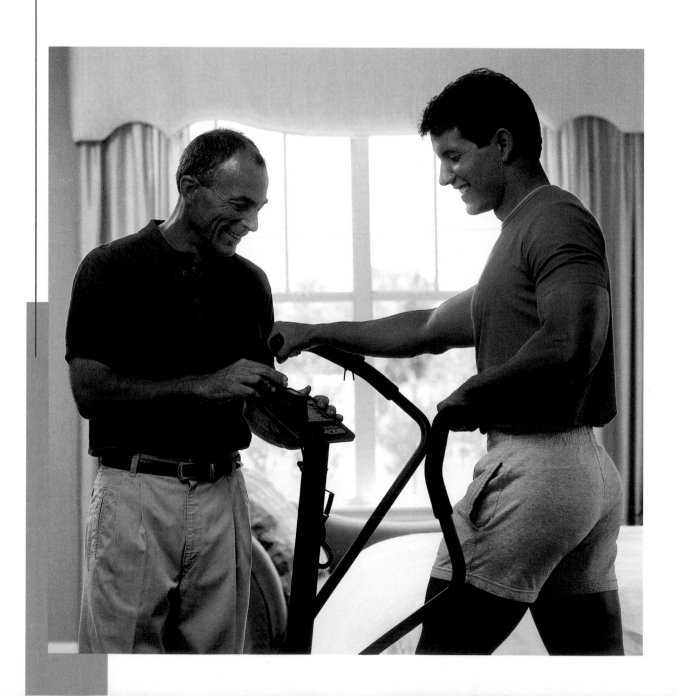

disease occur in childhood, parents can help children by demonstrating and practicing healthy eating. What kids learn at home, they most often practice when on their own.

KEYS TO HEART HEALTHY EATING

Americans on average consume 40 percent of their calories as fat calories. They eat enough meat, to be sure, but nibble at produce.

Ideally, you should reduce your saturated fat intake to 8 percent of total calories. This means consciously cutting back on marbled meats, high-fat dairy products and sweets made with lard or butter. Saturated fat really adds up when it is present in every meal, and most comfort foods are dense in fat. Reducing fat can be tough going at first. You need to be aware of what you are eating, every bite of every meal. When you identify excess fat, change the menu the next time.

Take advantage of the tastiness and healthy qualities in "good fats." Mono-unsaturated fats help reduce LDL cholesterol. Olive oil, canola oil, avocados, nuts, seeds and the fats in cold-water fish are heart-healthy, as long as you don't exceed the daily limit of 30 percent total calories from fat.

Adapt your menus to incorporate cold-water fish, walnuts, flaxseed and canola oil for their omega-3 fatty acids, which help thin the blood.

Experiment with soy in all its forms. There is a soy food that fits your tastes. Try soy meat substitutes in soups and chilis. Soy milk is great on its own or in a smoothie or shake. Tofu is a versatile soy protein source that is a

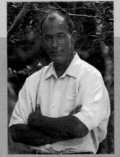

DR. RICHTER SAYS

Eating avocados, citrus, cranberries, fish, spinach and watermelon to consume mono-unsaturated fat, fiber, vitamin C, omega-3 fatty acids, lycopene, flavonoids, carotenoids, antioxidants and folate may help prevent heart disease, in some people.

staple in Asian cuisine. The fats and proteins in soy are great for your heart.

Bump up your intake of whole fruits and vegetables, which may stabilize your LDL cholesterol. Bring two or three pieces of fruit to work each day. Let your body teach you to be full from the natural bulk in whole fruits. When you do, you'll eat fewer rich lunches or desserts during the workday.

HAVE A PLAN

Eating well comes down to planning. With today's busy families and job conflicts, it may be easier to plan your nutrients around 21 meals per week, instead of three per day. With proper

planning, you can buy fresh produce for the family for a week and only go shopping once! By planning for a full week, you can build in social outings by "making up" for the big meal with a simple, yet satisfying, dinner the

next night. For example, a "continental" meal of fruit, bread dipped in herbed olive oil and low-fat soft cheese requires no cooking and is tasty and filling.

Think about what you eat every day. When the fast-food restaurant beckons, find an alternative. Stop the car, walk into the market and buy an apple. Better yet, buy a bag for your family.

cancer prevention
agenda

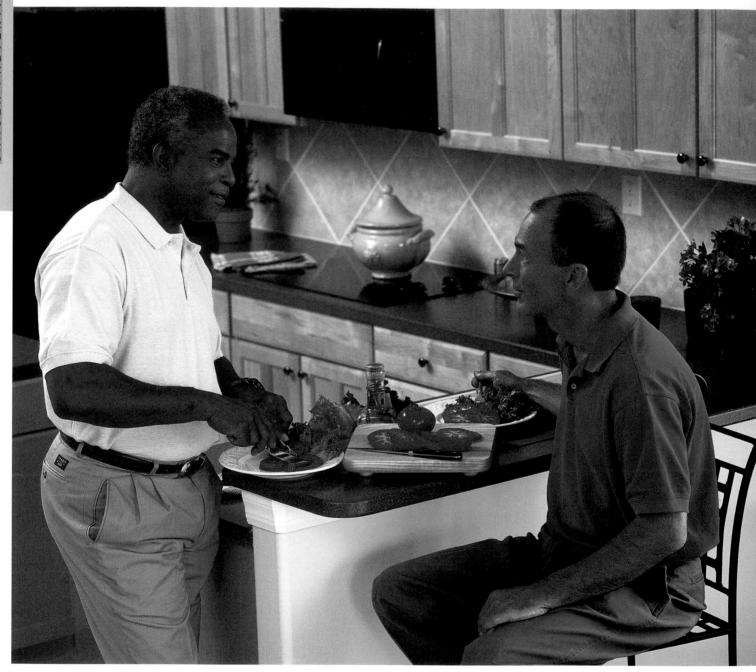

CANCER PREVENTION AND FOOD

Cancer prevention is foremost on most minds. People read tantalizing newspaper and magazine articles seeking new ways to prevent this dreaded disease. Is it possible to eat your way to this goal?

Physicians studying this complex subject cannot identify a single food or substance that will prevent cancer. But research supports this book's recommendations. Societies with high fiber consumption have lower rates of colon cancer than industrialized countries. Consumption of fruit and vegetables is associated with lower

Many supplements are marketed to prevent cancer, yet there is no evidence that any of them work. Spend your money instead on fresh, wholesome foods.

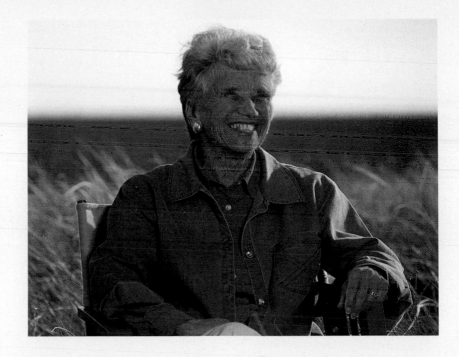

rates of lung, prostate, bladder, esophagus and stomach cancers. Diets low in fat also seem to help prevent cancers of the breast, colon and prostate.

Exactly why can eating an adequate amount of fruit and vegetables, and reducing fat intake help prevent cancer? Certainly the consumption of a variety of plant-based foods, with the antioxidants they contain, seems part of the answer. Also, fat in the diet may generally increase the metabolism of hormones that affect the breast, prostate and other organs. Cholesterol is the basic building block of estrogen and testosterone, so there might be a clue here. But overwhelmingly, obesity itself is associated with cancer. So reducing fat intake to lower your body weight should be a goal. In short, cancer prevention is most likely if you base your eating habits on fruit, vegetables and grains and limit your fat intake to substantially below 30 percent of total calories.

Today, many supplements are marketed to prevent cancer, yet there is no evidence that any of them work. Spend your money instead on fresh, wholesome foods. Exercise, avoid smoking and drink no more than one or two alcohol drinks daily. Finally, love yourself and your family, and teach them what you have learned about healthy eating. Offer your children a good example of how to eat well for their lifetimes.

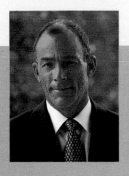

DR. RICHTER SAYS

Eating broccoli, cabbage, cantaloupe, cauliflower, garlic, grapefruit, grapes, onions, oranges, sweet potatoes, raspberries and tomatoes for vital phytonutrients and antioxidants may help prevent certain types of cancer.

menopausal menu

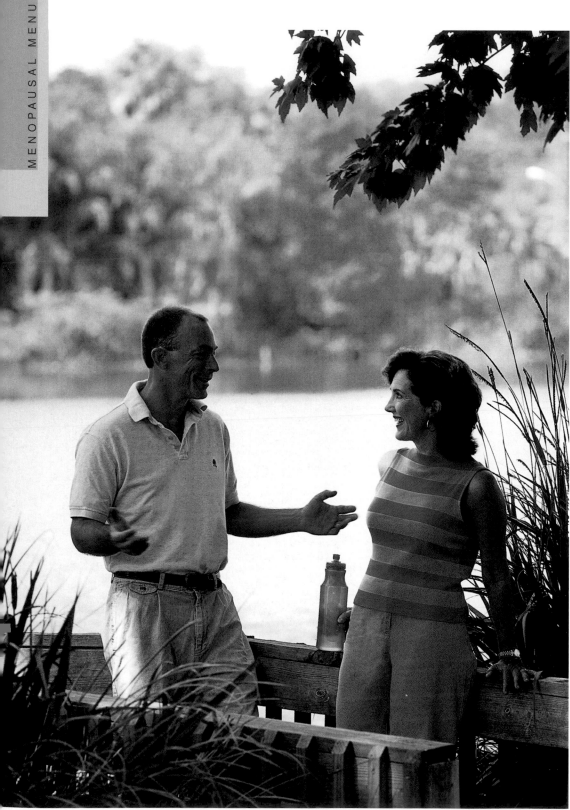

MENOPAUSE IS A TIME OF TRANSITION FOR women (and probably their husbands and families, too!). Other than pregnancy, there is no other time in a woman's life when nature can unsettle her with so much change. Both the body and emotions beat at a pace of their own. Some of the changes can be uncomfortable. Above all, they signify the beginning of a new life, full of opportunity and challenges. After all, if your menopause begins between 45 and 55, as it most often does, then you may anticipate 30 or more years of zestful life. Retirement and "empty nesting" leave you time to enjoy the things you want to do.

ENJOY THE OPTIONS

You have many options to help you reach your goals for this new chapter of your life. Start with eating well. Eat a diet with adequate fiber, for colon health. Soluble fiber decreases

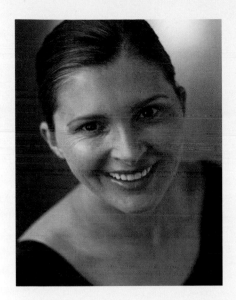

cholesterol. Fruit and vegetables are loaded with the latter, as are unrefined grains like oats, barley and cornmeal. Try to incorporate servings of beans (legumes) into your weekly fare. Many fruit and vegetables are packed not only with low-density carbohydrates, vitamins and minerals, but also with phytonutrients and antioxidants that may provide benefits for heart health, aging, dementia, memory and menopausal symptoms.

Soy is thought to be so beneficial for women's health that you should make a special effort to add it to your diet. One cup of tofu has about as much calcium as a cup of milk. Fresh soybeans are delicious and are available in today's produce

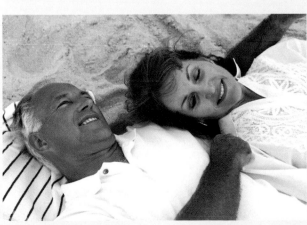

departments. If soy seems unpalatable, add soy powder to smoothies. You won't taste it, but you'll receive its benefits.

Soy isoflavones are "phytoestrogens" which may be beneficial for your heart, in relieving menopausal symptoms, and in possibly protecting against breast and uterine cancer. Soy is rather "dense" in calories, so pay attention to portions if you are watching your weight. However, these calories are amazingly good for you. The isoflavones are protein, which soy has in abundance, and the fats are mostly unsaturated, which help lower cholesterol levels.

Women may also enjoy bonus health benefits when they eat "cruciferous" vegetables like broccoli, cauliflower and Brussels sprouts. The phytonutrients in these foods seem to have cancer-protective qualities for women, just like soy, and are rich in fiber and vitamin C as well.

In fact, it is now easier than ever to consume nutrients without using supplements. Calcium-fortified orange juice, for

example, will make a big dent toward meeting your daily vitamin C and calcium requirements. Learn to ask, "what's in this?" when making your grocery list. Carefully selecting whole foods may fill your vitamin, mineral and fiber needs. Look at the labels on prepared food to properly gauge your intake of fat, salt and extra calories.

Don't forget to add exercise for a well-rounded approach to health. Even if you have never made any effort to exercise, see if it doesn't add to the quality of your next 30 years. Walking will increase your endurance,

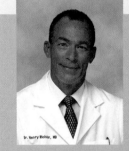

DR. RICHTER SAYS

Consider incorporating more soy into your diet. Eating apples, broccoli and grapes may boost your heart and digestive tract health.

fight osteoporosis and add muscle tissue that helps metabolize food faster and more efficiently.

Finally, you may want to consider herb therapy. Black cohash and plant-derived progesterone cream help to relieve hot flashes in some women. Flaxseed may thin blood and prevent strokes.

Enjoy your mature years. Just take some small steps for health, and you're on your way!

senior/anti-aging menu

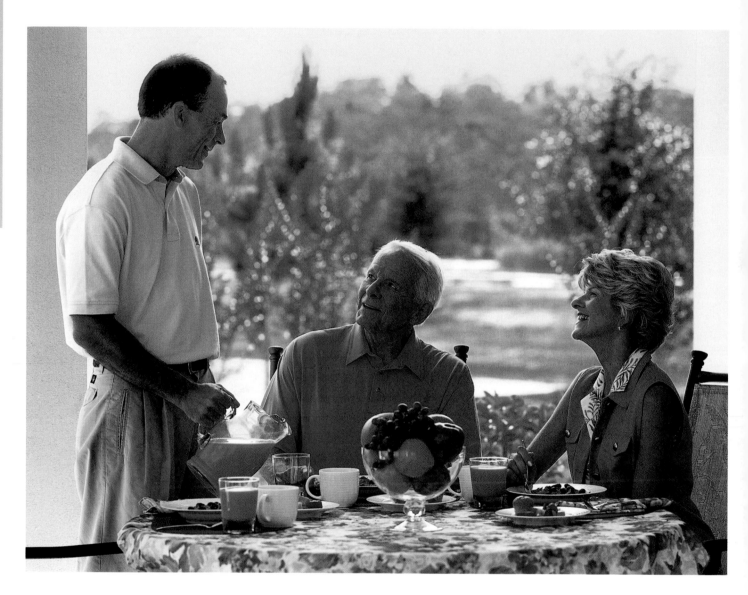

SENIORS: FEELING ACTIVE, GROWING YOUNG

SENIORS HAVE A LOT TO LIVE for. Having raised their families, they look forward to enjoying the rest of their lives. They want to do the things they love: golf, tennis or other sports, travel and being with the grandkids. In short, they want to play. Who can blame them? They've worked so hard to get there!

But worry takes the fun out of play. And seniors do have worries, especially about their health. Many health conditions affect seniors more than younger age groups. Women are more concerned about breast cancer, men about prostate cancer. Age-related damage to the eyes, memory or joints may strike as early as 50. The risk of a disabling heart attack or stroke becomes greater every year, especially if factors like diabetes or obesity are not controlled. But there is good news as well. Sticking to the basics and taking advantage of modern nutritional and exercise advice may add up to years of trouble-free health.

Because seniors have a slower metabolism than younger folks, they generally need fewer calories. As the food consumed each day falls to 1,300 calories or less, it is difficult to achieve the recommended amount of micronutrients. The solution is two-fold. First make every calorie worth it. Empty calories such as sweets, pastries and alcohol should be enjoyed in moderation. Experiment with non-traditional meals like

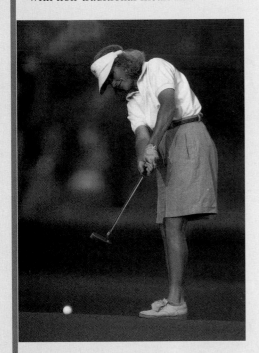

almond butter on whole wheat bread with fruit for breakfast.

Planning meals to be low in saturated fat is very important. High cholesterol is a major risk factor for hardening of the arteries, a cause of dementia and mini-strokes, which affect memory and balance. Whole grains, legumes and whole fruit and vegetables contain an abundance of nutrients with less potential for obesity than refined flours or milled (white) rice. The unsaturated fats in nuts and seeds are excellent natural blood thinners and

cholesterol reducers. Lean meats provide B vitamins. Dairy foods, fortified juice and produce provide the minerals calcium, potassium and magnesium to maintain normal blood pressure. (Yes, men need calcium, too!)

Medical research has outlined many potential benefits from eating whole foods. Fruit and vegetables, in particular, contain health-boosting phytonutrients. The phytoestrogens in soy and cruciferous vegetables may help boost bone strength, and may help ward off certain types of cancer. The great variety of antioxidants in produce possibly protect against blood vessel inflammation, which in turn reduce the risk of heart disease, stroke and decreased cognitive function. Early studies indicate that yellow or orange produce, brimming with colored carotenes, may lessen the risk of macular degeneration. Lycopene, found in tomatoes (and ketchup!) and watermelon, may be beneficial to men in preventing prostate disease.

Set a goal of eating five or more servings of fruit and vegetables daily before having dessert. Second, a vitamin and mineral supplement may provide added confidence. But do not go overboard! Too much of the fat-soluble vitamins (A, E, D, K) may be harmful and a physician can advise about vitamin therapy above the doses in a multi-vitamin.

An inactive body loses muscle before fat. Exercise is the ticket to strong muscles; it is the out-of-shape person who falls. Thus exercise complements

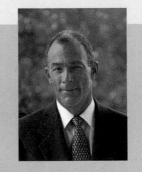

DR. RICHTER SAYS

Eating blueberries, cherries, citrus, kale, lemons, spinach, tomatoes and watermelon for a wealth of antioxidants may assist with memory, arthritis, cancer protection and heart health.

healthy eating for seniors. Getting the blood flowing hard every day will increase confidence, and let seniors wake up each morning eagerly and enthusiastically awaiting the day's fun.

produce shopping list

USE THIS LIST AS A GENERAL REFERENCE WHEN YOU SHOP. IF YOU HAVE A VARIETY OF FRESH produce on hand, it makes it easier to add to your favorite dishes during the week. It's like a traditional wardrobe...with a full closet, you can easily mix and match. So, shop wisely and eat well.

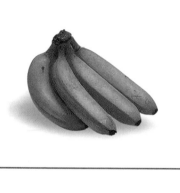

BANANAS
slice and add to cereal or take along whole for a midday snack

BERRIES
stir into yogurt, add to smoothies, make sorbet or top off waffles or cereal

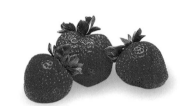

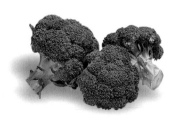

BROCCOLI
chop for pasta dishes, stir-frys or rice mixes, add to rice during last few minutes of cooking

CARROTS
use as a midday snack dipper, add to salads, steam as a side dish or chop into rice mixes

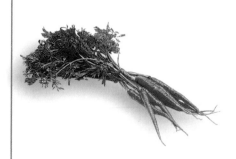

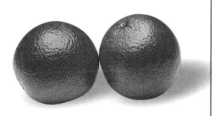

CITRUS
juice and drink, add to salads or use to marinate chicken breasts or seafood

LETTUCE & GREENS
tear up for a salad—worth two servings—and keep extra for sandwiches

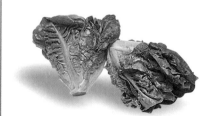

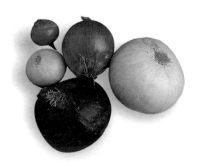

ONIONS
add to salads, stir-frys, pot roasts or slice onto sandwiches & burgers

TOMATOES
dash with vinaigrette for a European treat, or add to salads and sandwiches

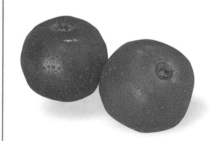

O GET SERIOUS ABOUT PRODUCE consumption, eat lots of fruit and vegetables daily. Each group contains different properties or phytochemicals that have unique effects on the human body. See how easy it is to get to five?

The next pages review the 40 most popular fruit and vegetables, according to the FDA's volume figures. Offering great taste, versatility and key nutrition, it's no wonder these are best-sellers!

TOP 20 FRUIT: Apple, Avocado, Banana, Cantaloupe, Cherry, Grapefruit, Grape, Honeydew Melon, Kiwifruit, Lemon, Lime, Nectarine, Orange, Peach, Pear, Pineapple, Plum, Strawberry, Tangerine and Watermelon.

TOP 20 VEGETABLES: Asparagus, Bell Pepper, Broccoli, Cabbage, Carrot, Cauliflower, Celery, Corn, Cucumber, Green Beans, Green Scallions, Lettuce, Leaf Lettuce, Mushrooms, Onion, Potato, Radish, Summer Squash/Zucchini, Sweet Potato and Tomato.

THE NATIONAL CANCER INSTITUTE'S FIVE POINTS TO REMEMBER FOR BETTER HEALTH

"Eat at least five servings of fruit and vegetables every day!"

"Eat at least one fruit, vegetable or juice that is high in vitamin A every day—such as sweet potatoes, carrots, spinach, dried apricots or winter squash."

"Eat at least one fruit, vegetable or juice that is high in vitamin C every day—such as snow peas, all citrus, pineapples or broccoli."

"Eat at least one high-fiber fruit or vegetable every day—such as apples, grapefruit, peas, papaya or beans."

"Eat cabbage family (cruciferous) vegetables several times a week—such as Brussels sprouts, cabbage, cauliflower or kale."

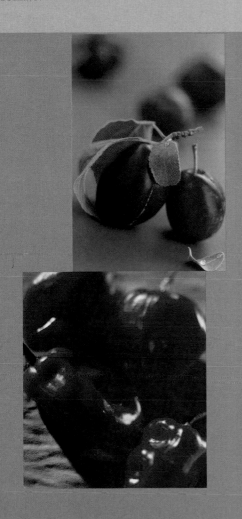

top 20 fruit

TOP 20 FRUIT

apple

HEALTH BENEFITS:
Excellent source of fiber.

SELECTION/STORAGE: Look for firm, smooth-skinned apples free of bruises and gouges. A dry brown patch on the skin (scald) does not affect the taste. Apple should have a fresh, not musty, smell. Store in a plastic bag in the refrigerator crisper or drawer away from vegetables.

PREPARATION/COOKING TIPS: To keep cut apples from browning, toss with citrus or apple juice, or dip in acidulated water.

VARIETIES/BEST USES: Braeburn (fresh eating, baking), Cameo® (fresh eating), Fuji (fresh eating, baking, salads), Gala (fresh eating), Granny Smith (fresh eating, pies), Jonagold (fresh eating, cooking), McIntosh (fresh eating), Pink Lady® (fresh eating, baking), Red Delicious (fresh eating), Rome Beauty (pies and applesauce).

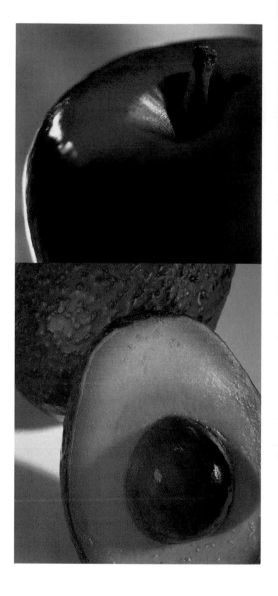

avocado

HEALTH BENEFITS: Cholesterol-free, sodium-free. Contains vitamin E.

SELECTION/STORAGE: A ripe avocado yields to gentle pressure. To speed the ripening process, place avocados in a paper bag with an apple. Poke a few holes in the bag and store at room temperature. California avocados change color from green to purple-black.

PREPARATION/COOKING TIPS: Slice in half and remove one side. Stick a fork in the large pit and twist to remove. Avocados discolor quickly, so rub lemon juice on the surface or cut just before serving.

VARIETIES/BEST USES: Florida (1/2 the fat and 2/3 the calories), Hass (guacamole).

NUTRITION FACTS

		SERVING SIZE	CALORIES	PROTEIN	FAT	CARBOHYDRATE	DIETARY FIBER	SODIUM
apple	UNITED STATES	1 med. w/skin	80	0g	0g	22g	5g	0mg
	VITAMINS/ MINERALS	A 53mcg, C 5mg, Calcium 7mg, Magnesium 5mg			ANTIOXIDANT	Carotenoids 30 mcg		

		SERVING SIZE	CALORIES	PROTEIN	FAT	CARBOHYDRATE	DIETARY FIBER	SODIUM
avocado	UNITED STATES	1/10 med.	35	0g	2.5g	3g	3g	0g
	VITAMINS/ MINERALS	A 612mcg, C 8mg, Folate 62mcg Magnesium 39mg, Potassium 599mg			ANTIOXIDANT	Alpha Carotenoids 28mcg, Beta Cryptoxanthin 36mcg, Lutein, Beta Carotenoids 53mcg		

Source: USDA-NCC Carotenoid Database for U.S. Foods

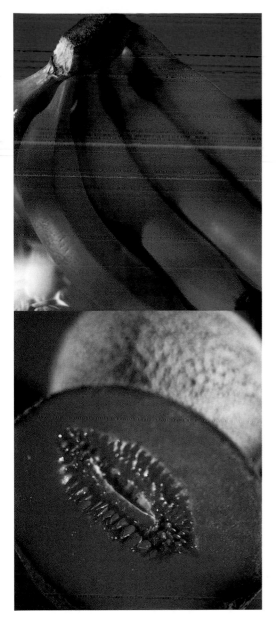

banana

HEALTH BENEFITS: Good source of potassium.

SELECTION/STORAGE: Select plump, evenly colored bananas. Brown speckles indicate ripeness. Store at room temperature. Refrigerate green plantains, keep yellow to black plantains at cool room temperature, out of the sun and well-ventilated. Store plantains away from other fruit.

PREPARATION/COOKING TIPS: If baking with bananas, choose slightly over-ripe fruit. Over-ripe bananas also great for frozen drinks. Can be frozen in an airtight bag with 1 teaspoon lemon juice for up to six months.

VARIETIES/BEST USES: Banana (fresh eating), Burro, Manzano (flambes and fritters), Nino (baking), Plantains (cooking).

cantaloupe

HEALTH BENEFITS: High in vitamin A and vitamin C.

SELECTION/STORAGE: Cantaloupes picked before they mature never reach full flavor. Check the stem end for a clean, smooth indentation, known as a "full-slip." If the edge is jagged, the cantaloupe was picked before maturity. A good melon is symmetrical and the blossom end gives with slight pressure. Avoid over-ripe melons with lumps or soft spots. Cantaloupes become more yellow as they ripen. Store ripe in the refrigerator for up to five days.

PREPARATION/COOKING TIPS: Slice cantaloupe in half. Scrape seeds out. Cantaloupe halves may be eaten with a spoon. Cantaloupe with prosciutto is a favorite appetizer or snack.

NUTRITION FACTS

banana		SERVING SIZE	CALORIES	PROTEIN	FAT	CARBOHYDRATE	DIETARY FIBER	SODIUM
	UNITED STATES	1 med.	110	1g	0g	29g	4g	0mg
	VITAMINS/ MINERALS	A 81mg, C 9mg, Folate 19mcg, Magnesium 29mcg, Potassium 396mg			ANTIOXIDANT	Alpha Carotenoids 5mcg, Beta Carotenoids 21mcg		

cantaloupe		SERVING SIZE	CALORIES	PROTEIN	FAT	CARBOHYDRATE	DIETARY FIBER	SODIUM
	UNITED STATES	1/4 med.	56	1g	0g	16g	1g	25mg
	VITAMINS/ MINERALS	A 3224mcg, C 42mg, Potassium 309mg			ANTIOXIDANT	Alpha Carotenoids 27mcg, Beta Carotenoids 1,595mcg, Lutein/Zeaxanthin 40mcg		

Source: USDA-NCC Carotenoid Database for U.S. Foods

top 20 fruit

cherry

HEALTH BENEFITS: Good source of vitamin C.

SELECTION/STORAGE: Look for firm, plump cherries with green stems. Keep cherries in a plastic bag in the refrigerator for two to three days. Cherries may be frozen for up to one year. Rinse and dry cherries and place in zip-seal plastic bag.

Close all but one inch, insert straw and suck out air; then fully seal.

PREPARATION/COOKING TIPS: Pit cherries with a cherry pitter or with the tip of a vegetable peeler. Add a few drops of pure almond extract to baked cherries to intensify cherry taste.

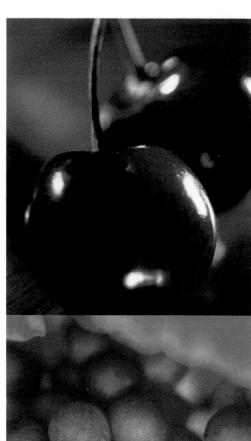

grape

HEALTH BENEFITS: Low-fat.

SELECTION/STORAGE: Grapes are picked and sold when ripe; they will not ripen further after picking. Look for firm, plump grapes firmly attached to flexible, not dry, stems. Discard over-ripe grapes, and refrigerate, unwashed, for no more than one week.

PREPARATION/COOKING TIPS: Wash grapes thoroughly before use. Remove from stems and eat out-of-hand, or add to salads, gelatins, yogurt or more. Ideally served at 60°, grapes are also a treat when frozen.

VARIETIES: Champagne, Concord, Green, Red, Seedless.

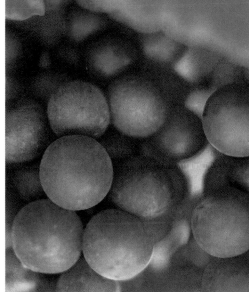

NUTRITION FACTS

cherry		SERVING SIZE	CALORIES	PROTEIN	FAT	CARBOHYDRATE	DIETARY FIBER	SODIUM
	UNITED STATES	1 cup	90	2g	0g	22g	3g	0mg
	VITAMINS/ MINERALS	A 1,283mg, C 10mg, Calcium 16mg, Potassium 173mg, Magnesium 9mg		ANTIOXIDANT		Carotenoids 28mcg		

grape		SERVING SIZE	CALORIES	PROTEIN	FAT	CARBOHYDRATE	DIETARY FIBER	SODIUM
	UNITED STATES	1 1/4 cups	90	1g	1g	24g	1g	0mg
	VITAMINS/ MINERALS	A 100 mcg, Calcium 14mg, Magnesium 5mg		ANTIOXIDANT		Carotenoids 39mcg, Ellagic Acid		

Source: USDA-NCC Carotenoid Database for U.S. Foods

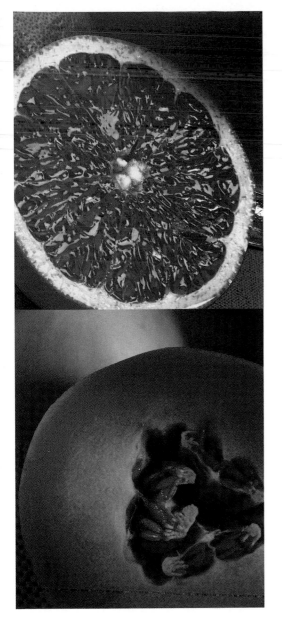

grapefruit

HEALTH BENEFITS: High in fiber and vitamin C.

SELECTION/STORAGE: Choose heavy fruit with smooth, thin skins. Grapefruit will not ripen after picking. Grapefruit can be kept at room temperature for six days, but keeps several weeks if refrigerated.

PREPARATION/COOKING TIPS: Peel or cut into wedges or slices. Grapefruit is juicier if rolled between your palm and the countertop a few seconds before eating. To remove pith easily, drop the whole grapefruit in boiling water. Remove from heat and let sit for four minutes. When you peel the grapefruit, the pith should come off with the skin.

honeydew melon

HEALTH BENEFITS: Excellent source of vitamin C.

SELECTION/STORAGE: Melons picked before maturity never reach full flavor. A good melon is symmetrical, the blossom end gives with slight pressure and the skin's surface has a slight wrinkling. Avoid rock-hard melons and over-ripe melons with lumps or soft spots. Refrigerate in a plastic bag up to five days.

PREPARATION/COOKING TIPS: Slice in half. With a spoon, scrape out the seeds. Slice halves into four or more pieces, then slice between the whitish-green flesh and the deeper-green rind. Honeydew should not be cooked.

NUTRITION FACTS

grapefruit		SERVING SIZE	CALORIES	PROTEIN	FAT	CARBOHYDRATE	DIETARY FIBER	SODIUM
	UNITED STATES	1 med.	60	1g	0g	15g	1g	0mg
	VITAMINS/ MINERALS	A 124 mcg, C 34mg, Calcium 12mg, Potassium 139mg,			ANTIOXIDANT	Alpha Carotenoids 5mcg, Beta Carotenoids 603mcg, Beta Cryptoxanthin 12mcg, Lutein/Zeaxanthin 13mcg, Lycopene 1,462mcg		

honeydew melon		SERVING SIZE	CALORIES	PROTEIN	FAT	CARBOHYDRATE	DIETARY FIBER	SODIUM
	UNITED STATES	1/10 med.	50	1g	0g	13g	1g	35mg
	VITAMINS/ MINERALS	A 40mcg, C 25mg, Potassium 271mg			ANTIOXIDANT	No government data		

Source: USDA-NCC Carotenoid Database for U.S. Foods

top 20 fruit

kiwifruit

HEALTH BENEFITS: Leading source of vitamin C.

SELECTION/STORAGE: Choose fruit with unbroken, unbruised skin. A ripe kiwifruit yields to gentle pressure. Most kiwis are sold hard and must be ripened at home. Ripen at room temperature, out of the sun. Refrigerate ripe kiwifruit for up to one week.

PREPARATION/COOKING TIPS: Scoop out with a spoon. Kiwifruit will not discolor when exposed to air and are a perfect choice for salads or garnish. Peel skin with a sharp knife or a vegetable peeler. Slice crosswise. Heating is not recommended.

VARIETIES: Green, Gold.

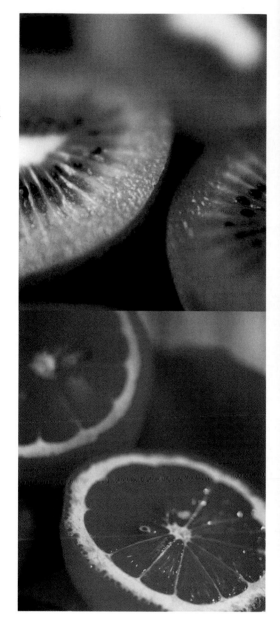

lemon

HEALTH BENEFITS: High in vitamin C.

SELECTION/STORAGE: Choose bright yellow, thin-skinned lemons. (For candied lemon peel, choose thicker-skinned lemons.) Lemons can be refrigerated for up to three weeks and leftover lemon juice should be frozen as refrigerated juice loses flavor faster.

PREPARATION/COOKING TIPS: One medium lemon yields two to three teaspoons of zest and three tablespoons of juice. To release more juice, place your palm on top of a room temperature lemon and roll it slowly, but firmly, across the countertop. Six medium lemons produce one cup of juice.

VARIETIES: Meyer (in baking or lemonade).

NUTRITION FACTS

kiwifruit		SERVING SIZE	CALORIES	PROTEIN	FAT	CARBOHYDRATE	DIETARY FIBER	SODIUM
	UNITED STATES	2 med.	100	2g	1g	24g	4g	0mg
	VITAMINS/ MINERALS	C 98mg, Calcium 26mg, Folate 38mcg, Magnesium 30mg, Potassium 332mg			ANTIOXIDANT	Carotenoids 28mcg, Lutein		

lemon		SERVING SIZE	CALORIES	PROTEIN	FAT	CARBOHYDRATE	DIETARY FIBER	SODIUM
	UNITED STATES	1 med.	15	0g	0g	5g	1g	5mg
	VITAMINS/ MINERALS	A 29 mcg, C 53mg, Calcium 26mg, Potassium 138mg			ANTIOXIDANT	Alpha Carotenoids 27mcg, Beta Carotenoids 1,595mcg, Lutein/Zeaxanthin 40mcg, Lycopene 1,462mcg		

Source: USDA-NCC Carotenoid Database for U.S. Foods

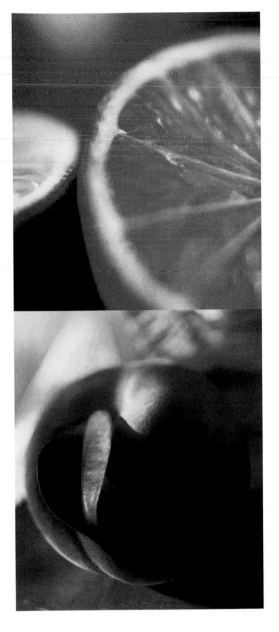

lime

HEALTH BENEFITS: High in vitamin C.

SELECTION/STORAGE: Select brightly colored, smooth-skinned, heavy limes. Some limes have small brown patches on their skin (russeting), but this does not affect flavor. Avoid hard or shriveled limes. Store limes in the refrigerator for up to 10 days.

PREPARATION/COOKING TIPS: To release more juice place your palm on the lime and roll it slowly across the countertop. Slice in half. Stick a fork into the fruit of the lime and twist back and forth to release juice. Six medium limes will yield about a half-cup of juice.

nectarine

HEALTH BENEFITS: Good source of vitamin C.

SELECTION/STORAGE: Avoid nectarines with soft spots or wrinkled skin. Ripen at room temperature, or place in a paper bag. When ripe, a nectarine is fragrant and yields slightly to the touch. Ripe nectarines may be refrigerated up to five days.

PREPARATION/COOKING TIPS: Nectarines don't need to be peeled before eating. They are an excellent substitution for strawberries in a shortcake recipe. Nectarines are good fresh or as a cooking fruit.

NUTRITION FACTS

lime		SERVING SIZE	CALORIES	PROTEIN	FAT	CARBOHYDRATE	DIETARY FIBER	SODIUM
	UNITED STATES	1 med.	20	0g	0g	7g	2g	0mg
	VITAMINS/ MINERALS	C 29 mg, Calcium 33mg, Potassium 102mg			ANTIOXIDANT	No government data		

nectarine		SERVING SIZE	CALORIES	PROTEIN	FAT	CARBOHYDRATE	DIETARY FIBER	SODIUM
	UNITED STATES	1 med.	70	1g	0g	16g	2g	0mg
	VITAMINS/ MINERALS	A 716 mcg, Potassium 212 mg			ANTIOXIDANT	Beta Carotenoids 101mcg, Beta Cryptoxanthin 59mcg		

Source: USDA-NCC Carotenoid Database for U.S. Foods

top 20 fruit

o r a n g e

HEALTH BENEFITS: High in fiber and vitamin C.

SELECTION/STORAGE: Pick oranges that are firm and heavy for their size. Russeting, a rough brown spot on the skin, does not affect the flavor. Ripe oranges may show a slight greening. Refrigerate or store at room temperature for up to two weeks.

PREPARATION/COOKING TIPS: Oranges are best eaten raw. Peel or cut into wedges or slices. If you choose a seeded variety, remove seeds before eating.

VARIETIES/BEST USES: Navel (fresh eating), Blood (in salads), Temple (fresh eating), Juice (juicing), Valencias (juicing).

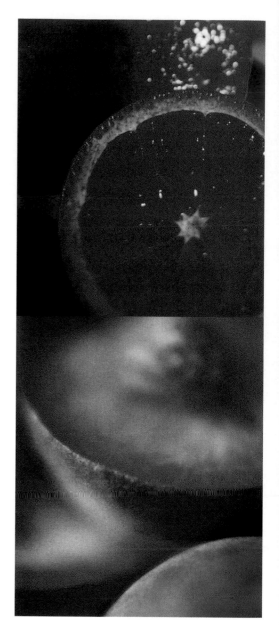

p e a c h

HEALTH BENEFITS: Good source of vitamin C.

SELECTION/STORAGE: The background color should be overall creamy or yellow. Peaches with a green background will not ripen further. Buy peaches with unbruised and unwrinkled skin. Ripen at room temperature in a paper bag. When soft to the touch and fragrant, peaches

may be stored, unwashed, in the refrigerator for up to two weeks. If brown spots appear, simply cut them off prior to eating.

PREPARATION/COOKING TIPS: Remove from the refrigerator one hour before eating. Wash peaches and gently rub them with a towel to remove the fuzziness. The flavor intensifies when warm.

NUTRITION FACTS

orange		SERVING SIZE	CALORIES	PROTEIN	FAT	CARBOHYDRATE	DIETARY FIBER	SODIUM
	UNITED STATES	1 med.	70	1g	0g	21g	7g	0mg
	VITAMINS/ MINERALS	A 205 mcg, C 53mg, Calcium 40mg, Folate 30mcg, Potassium 181mg			ANTIOXIDANT	Alpha Carotenoids 16mcg, Beta Carotenoids 51mcg, Lutein/Zeaxanthin 187mcg, Beta Cryptoxanthin 122mcg		

peach		SERVING SIZE	CALORIES	PROTEIN	FAT	CARBOHYDRATE	DIETARY FIBER	SODIUM
	UNITED STATES	1 med.	40	1g	0g	10g	2g	0mg
	VITAMINS/ MINERALS	A 535 mcg, Potassium 197mg			ANTIOXIDANT	Alpha Carotenoids 1mcg, Beta Carotenoids 97mcg, Beta Cryptoxanthin 24mcg, Lutein/Zeaxanthin 57mcg		

Source: USDA-NCC Carotenoid Database for U.S. Foods

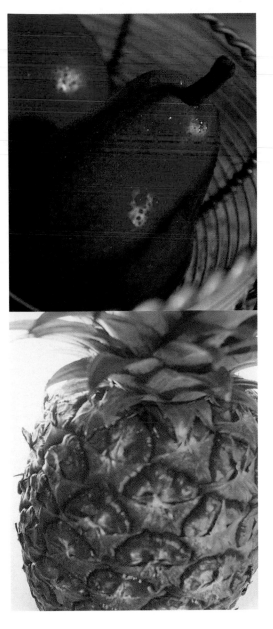

pear

HEALTH BENEFITS: Good source of fiber.

SELECTION/STORAGE: Pears bruise easily. Look for firm, unmarked and unbruised fruit. Pears ripen at room temperature. To hasten this process, place pears in a pierced paper bag with an apple or banana. Store ripe pears in a plastic bag in the refrigerator for up to five days.

PREPARATION/COOKING TIPS: Wash ripe pears and gently dry. Remove skin before cooking.

VARIETIES/BEST USES: Anjou (cooking), Asian, Bartlett, Bosc (fresh eating), Comice (not cooked), Forelle, Packham (fresh eating), Seckel (canning and pickling), Taylor's Gold (fresh eating).

pineapple

HEALTH BENEFITS: High in vitamin C, fat-free

SELECTION/STORAGE: Choose a pineapple with crown leaves that are fresh and green. The pineapple itself should be fragrant, heavy and symmetrical in size. Once cut, tightly sealed pineapple can remain in the refrigerator for three more days.

PREPARATION/COOKING TIPS: Use pineapples as a dessert or snack, in salads, in drinks, in baking and in cooking. Cut a thick slice from the top and the bottom. Pare skin from the top downward. Next, remove the eyes by cutting diagonal grooves. Finally, cut into eights and remove the core section from each.

VARIETIES: Del Monte™ Gold Extra Sweet, Del Monte™ Hawaii Gold and Champaka.

NUTRITION FACTS

pear		SERVING SIZE	CALORIES	PROTEIN	FAT	CARBOHYDRATE	DIETARY FIBER	SODIUM
	UNITED STATES	1 med.	98	1g	1g	25g	5g	0mg
	VITAMINS/ MINERALS	A 20mcg, C 4mg, Calcium 11mg, Potassium 125mg			ANTIOXIDANT	Alpha Carotenoids 6mcg, Beta Carotenoids 27mcg		

pineapple		SERVING SIZE	CALORIES	PROTEIN	FAT	CARBOHYDRATE	DIETARY FIBER	SODIUM
	UNITED STATES	2 slices 3″ diam. 3/4″ thick	60	1g	0g	16g	1g	10mg
	VITAMINS/ MINERALS	A 23mcg, C 15mg, Magnesium 14mg			ANTIOXIDANT	Beta Carotenoids 30mcg		

Source: USDA-NCC Carotenoid Database for U.S. Foods

top 20 fruit

plum

HEALTH BENEFITS: Good source of vitamin C.

SELECTION/STORAGE: Choose plums that give slightly to palm pressure. Avoid plums with soft spots or wrinkled skin. Ripen at room temperature, or place in a paper bag. Ripe plums can be placed in the refrigerator for up to five days.

PREPARATION/COOKING TIPS: Wash plums, cut in half and remove the pit. For an easy dessert, sauté quartered plums and brown sugar in a little butter until soft.

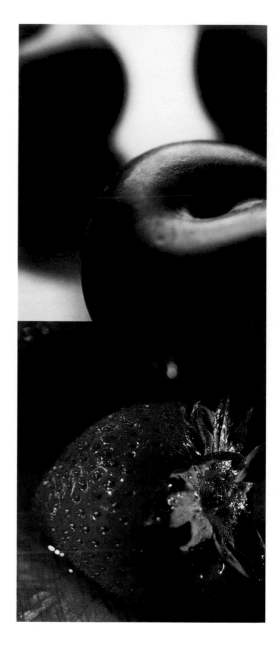

strawberry

HEALTH BENEFITS: High in vitamin C and contains fiber.

SELECTION/STORAGE: Look for brightly colored, plump berries with a strong scent. Small berries are the tastiest. Strawberries do not ripen after they have been picked. Do not wash before storing. Place in a single layer on a paper towel in a moisture-proof container. In the refrigerator, they will last two to three days.

PREPARATION/COOKING TIPS: Rinse berries thoroughly. With a small, sharp knife, remove the hull. To get maximum juice, slice strawberries and let sit at room temperature for two hours.

NUTRITION FACTS

		SERVING SIZE	CALORIES	PROTEIN	FAT	CARBOHYDRATE	DIETARY FIBER	SODIUM
plum	UNITED STATES	2 med.	91	1g	1g	21g	2.5g	0mg
	VITAMINS/ MINERALS	A 323 mcg, C 9mg, Magnesium 7mg, Potassium 172mg			ANTIOXIDANT	Beta Carotenoids 98mcg, Beta Cryptoxanthin 16mcg		

		SERVING SIZE	CALORIES	PROTEIN	FAT	CARBOHYDRATE	DIETARY FIBER	SODIUM
strawberry	UNITED STATES	8 med.	45	1g	0g	12g	4g	0mg
	VITAMINS/ MINERALS	A 27mcg, C 56mg, Folate 18mcg, Potassium 166mg		ANTIOXIDANT		Alpha Carotenoids 5mcg, Ellagic Acid		

Source: USDA-NCC Carotenoid Database for U.S. Foods

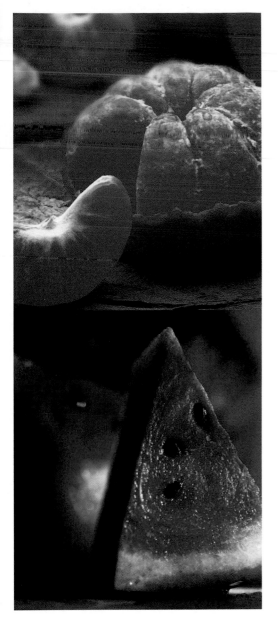

tangerine

HEALTH BENEFITS: High in vitamin C.

SELECTION/STORAGE: Choose tangerines that are plump and heavy for their size, as these will be juiciest. They should be soft, but firm to the touch. The color may vary from light to deep orange, but the skin should be glossy. Tangerines may be kept for up to one week in the refrigerator.

PREPARATION/COOKING TIPS: Tangerines are best eaten raw. If you must cook them, heat gently and do not boil or they will lose their flavor. Tangerines are good in salads, on custards or as side dishes with candied lemon zest.

watermelon

HEALTH BENEFITS: Excellent source of vitamin C.

SELECTION/STORAGE: Avoid melons with a flat side. The skin should be dull, not shiny. Slap the melon and listen for a hollow thump. Refrigerate for no more than a week.

PREPARATION/COOKING TIPS: Cut melon into circular slices. Most seeds are in concentric circles. Use cookie cutter to remove seedless center. With a sharp knife, remove the ring of seeds. Cut remaining ring at inner rind. Cube reserved fruit into one-inch cubes. Serve watermelon chunks tossed with orange juice, mint leaves, a little sugar and toasted almonds.

NUTRITION FACTS

tangerine

		SERVING SIZE	CALORIES	PROTEIN	FAT	CARBOHYDRATE	DIETARY FIBER	SODIUM
	UNITED STATES	1 med.	74	1g	0g	19g	4g	2mg
	VITAMINS/ MINERALS	A 920mcg, C 31mg, Calcium 14mg, Folate 20mg			ANTIOXIDANT	Alpha Carotenoids 14mcg, Beta Carotenoids 71mcg, Lutein/Zeaxanthin 243mcg, Beta Cryptoxanthin 485mcg		

watermelon

		SERVING SIZE	CALORIES	PROTEIN	FAT	CARBOHYDRATE	DIETARY FIBER	SODIUM
	UNITED STATES	1/18 med.	80	1g	0g	27g	2g	10mg
	VITAMINS/ MINERALS	A 366mcg, C 10mg, Magnesium 11mg			ANTIOXIDANT	Beta Carotenoids 295mcg, Lutein/Zeaxanthin 17mcg, Lycopene 4,868mcg, Beta Cryptoxanthin 103mcg		

Source: USDA-NCC Carotenoid Database for U.S. Foods

berries

They're beautiful in color, bursting with flavor and can turn desserts into delicious bites of pleasure. Recent studies show that in addition to all their natural good looks and taste,

	DESCRIPTION	TASTE	SELECTION
blackberry	Grow on bramble bushes. Bumpy, and purplish-black in color. The largest of wild berries.	Sweet & juicy.	Available May through September. Choose firm, plump, dark-colored; avoid those with mold.
black/red grape	Deep rose-pink to purple-black.	Most flavor resides in the skin. Juicy.	Choose plump, fragrant with a dusting of silver; avoid those browned at the stem.
blueberry	Wild berries are smaller than cultivated varieties.	Sweet & juicy.	Available May to October, US; year-round, Chile. Plump, firm, indigo-blue with a silvery frost; avoid wrinkled, dry, moldy.
boysenberry	A hybrid of raspberry & blackberry.	Tart, yet sweet.	Available May through August. Choose plump, firm, uniform in color; avoid those leaking or stained.
cranberry	Deep red, firm.	Tart, firm.	Available October through December. Choose dark-red; discard those shriveled, soft, discolored.
currant	Red, pink or white. Grown on deciduous shrubs. Related to gooseberry.	Tart.	Available June to August or, December to February. Choose tiny, glossy, translucent; avoid dried on the vine.
gooseberry	White, green or purple. Related to currant.	Distinctively tart. Pinkish-purple are less tart.	Available New Zealand, November to January; America, May to August. Choose firm, full. Somewhat fuzzy skin.
green grape	Usually white, the color varies from pale green to amber-yellow.	Clean, sweet. Most flavor resides in the skin.	Choose those that are plump, firmly attached to the stem; not browning.
loganberry	A cross between blackberry and raspberry, deep red.	Uniquely tart.	Available mid-June to mid-July. Choose those vibrant in color.
mulberry	Black, white or red. Botanically not a berry, this is a distant cousin of breadfruit. Grows on deciduous trees. In appearance to a swollen loganberry.	Refreshingly tart, as is grapefruit. Juicy. White are the sweetest.	Select succulent, full.
fuyu persimmon	Pale orange to brilliant orange, red. Tomato shaped with 4-leaf capped stem.	Sweet, combination of pumpkin, plum & honey, unlike most persimmons.	Available September through November and April through May. Select those that yield to gentle pressure.
hachiya persimmon	Deep orange, no trace of yellow. Acorn-shaped with 4-leaf capped stem.	Bitter until ripe.	Available September through November and April through May. Choose those softer than a baby's cheek, nearly liquid.
raspberry	Black, red or gold.	Sweet.	Available year-round. Peaks June through September. Choose fragrant, plumb, intensely colored without hulls; avoid those with mold.
strawberry	The inside-out berry…featuring its seeds on the outside. Bright red.	Sweet.	Available year-round. Peak: April to June. Select those brightly colored with a strong scent. Small berries usually are tastier.

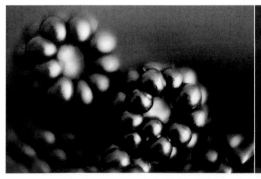 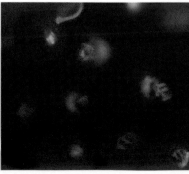 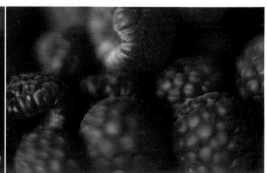

berries are abundant in antioxidants, so much so that they rank far above most other fruit and vegetables. If you need more incentive to munch, just remember that berries contain fiber, are low in calories and are virtually fat-free.

STORAGE	PREPARATION	USAGE	HEALTH TIP
Lay, single layer, on paper towel lined baking sheet. Cover with paper towel. Refrigerate for up to 2 days.	Do not wash until ready to use.	Jam, pies & cakes.	A sweet source of vitamin C and an overall good health promoter.
Refrigerate, unwashed, up to one week.	Do not wash until ready to use.	Jelly & juice.	Partake to possibly improve circulation and enhance memory.
Refrigerate tightly covered, up to one week.	Do not wash until ready to use.	Fruit salad, pies & muffins.	Maximum antioxidant resource. Optimum helper for age-related decline.
Lay, single layer, on paper towel-lined baking sheet. Cover with paper towel. Refrigerate for up to 2 days.	Do not wash until ready to use.	Fruit salad, jam, pie.	Source of fiber which maintains a healthy digestive tract.
Refrigerate, up to one month.	Do not wash until ready to use. Rinse thoroughly.	Relish/sauce, bread stuffing, juice. Dried on salads.	Possible chronic disease preventer, such as: cancer, stroke, heart.
Refrigerate, on a paper towel, in clusters, up to 3 days.	Do not wash until ready to use.	Fruit compote, jelly.	The pigment adds vibrance to the berry and to your bloodstream, as a cancer deterrent.
Refrigerate, up to 2 weeks.	Cut small tips and stems.	In purée.	May break down cancer-causing agents in the body.
Refrigerate, unwashed, up to 1 week.	Wash thoroughly.	Best when eaten raw.	May curb age-related effects.
Lay, single layer, on paper towel lined baking sheet. Cover with paper towel. Refrigerate for up to 2 days.	Do not wash until ready to use.	Pies & wines.	May lower "bad" cholesterol in the fight against heart disease.
Lay, single layer, on paper towel-lined baking sheet. Cover with paper towel. Refrigerate for up to 2 days.	Do not wash until ready to use.	Pies, tarts, wine or dried. Blend with apples or pears.	Packed with antioxidants that possibly affect blood clot formation for optimum heart health.
Store in a cool place and use within a month. Refrigerate ripe fruit up to 3 days.	Rinse, peel.	Fruit salads & desserts.	Keeps gums and teeth healthy and heals wounds…all due to vitamin C.
Use ripe Hachiyas within a few days. Refrigerate ripe fruit up to 3 days.	Rinse, peeling optional.	In desserts or canning.	Contains vitamin C for prevention of cataracts and the promotion of good vision.
Lay, single layer, on paper towel-lined baking sheet. Cover with paper towel. Refrigerate for up to 3 days.	Do not wash until ready to use.	Jam, pie, drinks, smoothies, parfait & sorbets.	Perhaps an exceptional cancer fighter!
Place single layer, on a paper towel, in a sealed container. Refrigerate up to 3 days.	Do not wash until ready to use. Remove the hull.	Jam, pie, salads, tarts, smoothies, parfait, on ice cream.	Ellagic acid carrier for possible cancer prevention.

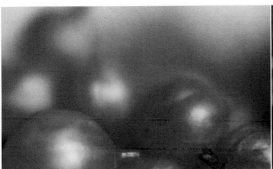
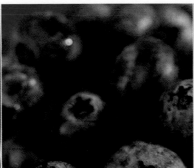
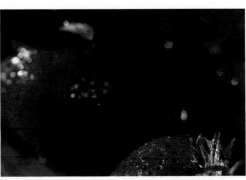

top 20 vegetables

asparagus

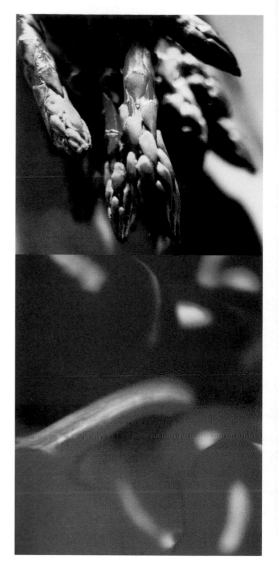

HEALTH BENEFIT: Excellent source of folate.

SELECTION/STORAGE: Buy firm, bright-green (NOT khaki) stalks with tight, purple-tinted buds. Use as soon as possible after purchase. To store, trim the ends. Stand stalks upright in one inch of water in a tall container. Cover the tops with a plastic bag and refrigerate for no more than a few days.

PREPARATION/COOKING TIPS: Gently snap each asparagus stalk at the bottom; it should break at the very spot where the woodiness begins. Discard woody ends. Soak in cold water. Peel thicker stalks.

green, red, yellow bell pepper

HEALTH BENEFIT: High in vitamin C.

SELECTION/STORAGE: Look for firm, vividly colored peppers with smooth and shiny skin. Check for soft spots. Refrigerate, wrapped in plastic, for up to two weeks.

PREPARATION/COOKING TIPS: Wash bell peppers well. With a paring knife, slice around the edge of the stem. Remove stem. Cut pepper in half; remove remaining seeds. Stuff, roast or use in salads, stir-frys and casseroles.

VARIETIES: Green, red, yellow.

NUTRITION FACTS

asparagus		SERVING SIZE	CALORIES	PROTEIN	FAT	CARBOHYDRATE	DIETARY FIBER	SODIUM
	UNITED STATES	5 spears	25	2g	0g	4g	2g	0mg
	VITAMINS/ MINERALS	A 583mcg, C 13mg, Calcium 21mg, Folate 128mg, Magnesium 18mg, Potassium 273mg			ANTIOXIDANT	Alpha Carotenoids 12mcg, Beta Carotenoids 493mcg		

bell pepper		SERVING SIZE	CALORIES	PROTEIN	FAT	CARBOHYDRATE	DIETARY FIBER	SODIUM
	UNITED STATES	1 med.	30	1g	0g	7g	2g	2mg
	VITAMINS/ MINERALS	Red: A 5700mcg, C 150mg, Calcium 9mg, Folate 22mcg, Magnesium 10mg, Potassium 177mg			ANTIOXIDANT	Green: Alpha Carotenoids 22mcg, Beta Carotenoids 198mcg Yellow: Beta Carotenoids 120mcg Red: Alpha Carotenoids 59mcg, Beta Carotenoids 2,379mcg, Beta Cryptoxanthin 2,205mcg		

Source: USDA-NCC Carotenoid Database for U.S. Foods

top 20 vegetables

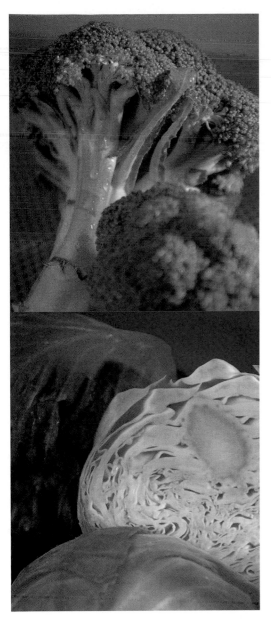

broccoli

HEALTH BENEFIT: Excellent source of vitamin C, fiber and folate. Also contains vitamin A. Member of cruciferous family.

SELECTION/STORAGE: Choose tightly formed, deep-green heads with firm stalks. Some varieties are tinged with purple. Yellowing heads are past their prime. Refrigerate in a perforated plastic bag for no more than four days.

PREPARATION/COOKING TIPS: Trim ends and peel the stalks. Always rinse broccoli in cold water before cooking. Cut the florets from the stalk in even sizes. Stir-fry, steam or puree. Try partially steamed broccoli sautéed with garlic and olives, or with ginger and sesame seeds.

cabbage

HEALTH BENEFIT: High in vitamin C. Member of cruciferous family.

SELECTION/STORAGE: Choose cabbages that are heavy for their size with crisp, tightly packed leaves. Tightly wrap in plastic and refrigerate for up to one week.

PREPARATION/COOKING TIPS: Cabbage can be eaten raw in salads and slaws. If boiling or steaming cabbage, cook until it's just tender. To avoid strong cooking odor, place a piece of bread, a walnut or a piece of parsley in the water.

VARIETIES/BEST USES: Red (slaws, salads), Chinese (stir-frys), Green (soups).

NUTRITION FACTS

broccoli		SERVING SIZE	CALORIES	PROTEIN	FAT	CARBOHYDRATE	DIETARY FIBER	SODIUM
	UNITED STATES	1 med. stalk	35	1g	0g	8g	2g	65mg
	VITAMINS/ MINERALS	A 1,542mcg, C 93mg, Calcium 48mg, Folate 71mcg, Magnesium 25mg, Potassium 325mg, Selenium 3mcg,			ANTIOXIDANT	Alpha Carotenoids 1mcg, Beta Carotenoids 779mcg, Lutein/Zeaxanthin 2,445mcg		

cabbage		SERVING SIZE	CALORIES	PROTEIN	FAT	CARBOHYDRATE	DIETARY FIBER	SODIUM
	UNITED STATES	1/12 head	25	1g	0g	5g	2g	20mg
	VITAMINS/ MINERALS	A 133mcg, C 32mg, Calcium 47mg, Folate 43mg, Magnesium 15mg, Potassium 246mg,			ANTIOXIDANT	Beta Carotenoids 65mcg, Lutein/Zeaxanthin 310mcg		

Source: USDA-NCC Carotenoid Database for U.S. Foods

top 20 vegetables

carrot

HEALTH BENEFIT: High in beta-carotene, precursor of vitamin A.

SELECTION/STORAGE: Choose long, narrow carrots for the best taste. Avoid carrots that are bendable, have cracks or show withering. If buying carrots with greens attached, remove them before refrigerating the carrots in a plastic bag. Do not store carrots next to apples.

PREPARATION/COOKING TIPS: Although carrots lose some of their vitamins when peeled, they taste better with skins removed. Freshen limp carrots in a bowl of ice water. Carrots can be shredded, julienned or cut into "coins" and cooked any number of ways.

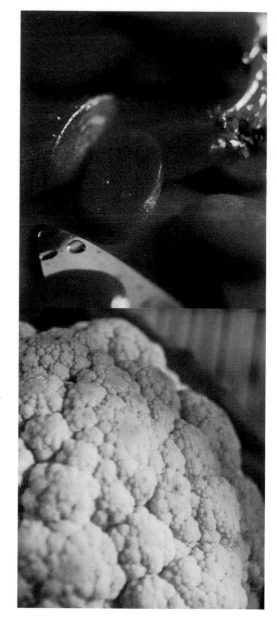

cauliflower

HEALTH BENEFIT: High in vitamin C. Member of cruciferous family.

SELECTION/STORAGE: Look for heads that are white, firm and heavy for their size with no speckling on the head or the leaves. Avoid cauliflower with brown patches. Refrigerate, tightly wrapped, for no more than five days.

PREPARATION/COOKING TIPS: Peel off stem leaves. Turn cauliflower upside down. Cut the stem just above where the florets join together. Separate the florets into equal sizes. Cut if necessary. Cauliflower is so versatile it can be eaten raw, blanched, steamed, boiled or fried.

NUTRITION FACTS

carrot

	SERVING SIZE	CALORIES	PROTEIN	FAT	CARBOHYDRATE	DIETARY FIBER	SODIUM
UNITED STATES	1 med. 7″ long	35	1g	0g	8g	2g	40mg
VITAMINS/ MINERALS	A 28,129mcg, C 9mg, Calcium 27mg, Folate 14mcg, Magnesium 15mg, Potassium 323mg			ANTIOXIDANT	Alpha Carotenoids 4,649mcg, Beta Carotenoids 8,836mcg		

cauliflower

	SERVING SIZE	CALORIES	PROTEIN	FAT	CARBOHYDRATE	DIETARY FIBER	SODIUM
UNITED STATES	1 med.	80	3g	1g	18g	3g	0mg
VITAMINS/ MINERALS	A 19mcg, C 46mg, Calcium 22mg, Folate 57mcg, Magnesium 15mg, Potassium 303mg			ANTIOXIDANT	Beta Carotenoids 65mcg, Lutein/Zeaxanthin 310mcg		

Source: USDA-NCC Carotenoid Database for U.S. Foods

top 20 vegetables

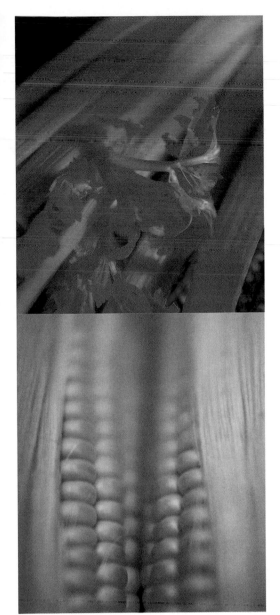

celery

HEALTH BENEFIT: High in vitamin C, fiber and folate. Also contains vitamin A. Member of cruciferous family.

SELECTION/STORAGE: Buy stalks that are firm and unblemished with leaves that are green, not yellow. Refrigerate in a plastic bag for up to two weeks.

PREPARATION/COOKING TIPS: Celery needs to be thoroughly cleaned. Pull ribs away from stalk and wash off dirt. If celery is tough, snap the rib near the top without breaking the strings and pull the piece towards the bottom. Do not discard leaves, but save for flavoring soups or pasta sauce. Eat celery raw, braised or baked.

corn

HEALTH BENEFIT: High in vitamin C.

SELECTION/STORAGE: Choose corn with husks that are tightly wrapped, grass-green and slightly damp. The corn silk can be dry, but not rotting, and stem ends moist, not yellowed. Do not store corn.

PREPARATION/COOKING TIPS: Shuck the corn (remove the husks and the corn silk) right before boiling. To roast or grill corn, pull the husks down (not off) the stem, remove the corn silk, rewrap husks and tie at the top. (Soak husked corn in water 10 minutes before grilling.)

NUTRITION FACTS

celery		SERVING SIZE	CALORIES	PROTEIN	FAT	CARBOHYDRATE	DIETARY FIBER	SODIUM
	UNITED STATES	2 med. stalks	13	0.5g	0g	3g	1g	70mg
	VITAMINS/ MINERALS	A 134mcg, C 7mg, Calcium 40mg, Folate 25mcg, Magnesium 11mg, Potassium 287mg			ANTIOXIDANT	Beta Carotenoids 150mcg, Lutein/Zeaxanthin 232mcg		

corn		SERVING SIZE	CALORIES	PROTEIN	FAT	CARBOHYDRATE	DIETARY FIBER	SODIUM
	UNITED STATES	1/6 head	25	2g	0g	5g	2g	30mg
	VITAMINS/ MINERALS	A 281mcg, C 7mg, Folate 46mcg, Magnesium 37mg, Potassium 270mg			ANTIOXIDANT	Beta Carotenoids 14mcg, Lutein/Zeathanin 1,800mcg (cooked)		

Source: USDA-NCC Carotenoid Database for U.S. Foods

top 20 vegetables

cucumber

HEALTH BENEFIT: Good source of vitamin C.

SELECTION/STORAGE: Choose firm, unblemished cucumbers. Avoid ones with soft spots and yellow streaks. Refrigerate unwashed in a plastic bag for up to one week.

PREPARATION/COOKING TIPS: Wash well or peel to remove the waxy coating. To remove seeds, slice in half lengthwise and drag a spoon through the seeds to remove them. Slice an inch from each end of the cucumber, as bitterness tends to gather there. Never cook cucumbers.

VARIETIES/BEST USES: Common, English/Burpless, Japanese, Kirby.

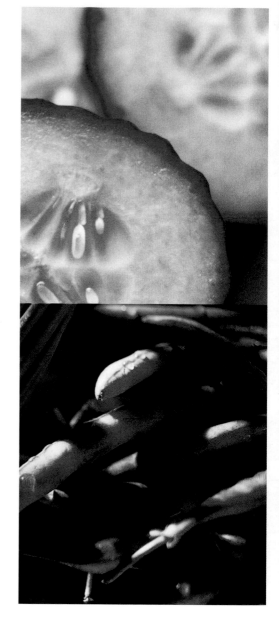

green beans

HEALTH BENEFIT: Good source of fiber.

SELECTION/STORAGE: Choose brightly colored beans with a smooth surface. Avoid those that are leathery or withered. If the bean can be bent at a 90° angle without snapping it, the bean is past its prime. Refrigerate, unwashed, in an airtight bag for up to four days.

PREPARATION/COOKING TIPS: Wash in cool water, drain and remove stems. Remove strings if necessary. The tip does not have to be trimmed. Drop beans in boiling, salted water for three minutes or until just tender.

VARIETIES: Pole, French, Yellow Wax.

NUTRITION FACTS

cucumber

	SERVING SIZE	CALORIES	PROTEIN	FAT	CARBOHYDRATE	DIETARY FIBER	SODIUM
UNITED STATES	1/3 med.	15	1g	0g	3g	1g	0mg
VITAMINS/ MINERALS	A 215mcg, C 5mg, Calcium 14mg, Folate 13mcg, Magnesium 11mg, Potassium 144mg			ANTIOXIDANT	Beta Carotenoids 138mcg		

green beans

	SERVING SIZE	CALORIES	PROTEIN	FAT	CARBOHYDRATE	DIETARY FIBER	SODIUM
UNITED STATES	3/4cup, cut	25	1g	0g	5g	3g	0mg
VITAMINS/ MINERALS	A 668mcg, C 16mg, K 209mg, Calcium 37mg, Folate 37mcg, Magnesium 25mg, Potassium 209mg			ANTIOXIDANT	Alpha Carotenoids 68mcg, Beta Carotenoids 377mcg, Lutein/Zeaxanthin 640mcg		

Source: USDA-NCC Carotenoid Database for U.S. Foods

top 20 vegetables

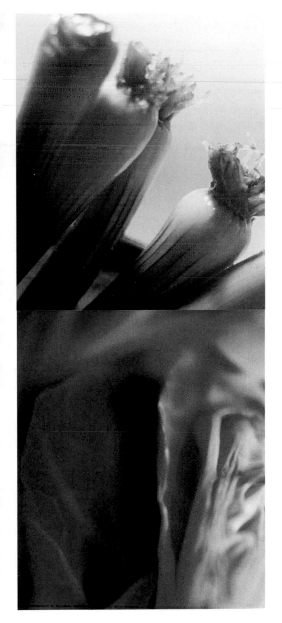

green onion

HEALTH BENEFIT: Low-fat.

SELECTION/STORAGE: Look for green onions and scallions with bright-green, crisp tops and firm white bases. Select those with the most white up the stem. Refrigerate, wrapped in a plastic bag, for up to five days.

PREPARATION/COOKING TIPS: Most of this vegetable is edible. Slice off the white roots at the base and then slice as desired. Many recipes will specify white part only, or white and inches of the green. Green onions are good in salads and they can be braised in butter and stock.

VARIETIES: Scallions, Leeks.

lettuce

HEALTH BENEFIT: Fat-free. Iceberg contains fewer vitamins than its darker green cousins.

SELECTION/STORAGE: Choose firm, densely packed heads that are heavy for their size. Avoid any that have browning or slimy edges. Refrigerate, unwashed, in a sealed plastic bag for up to two weeks.

PREPARATION/COOKING TIPS: Remove the core with a sharp knife or rap the core against the counter; then hold the core, twist it and lift out. Run water into the cavity until it flows up out of the leaves. Invert the lettuce head and drain. Rip lettuce leaves by hand.

NUTRITION FACTS

green onion

	SERVING SIZE	CALORIES	PROTEIN	FAT	CARBOHYDRATE	DIETARY FIBER	SODIUM
UNITED STATES	1 med.	10	0g	0.1g	2g	1g	5mg
VITAMINS/ MINERALS	A 55mcg, C 12mg, Calcium 59mg, Folate 64mg, Magnesium 28mg, Potassium 180mg			ANTIOXIDANT	Alpha Carotenoids 6mcg, Beta Carotenoids 391mcg		

lettuce

	SERVING SIZE	CALORIES	PROTEIN	FAT	CARBOHYDRATE	DIETARY FIBER	SODIUM
UNITED STATES	1/8 head	15	1g	0g	3g	1g	10mg
VITAMINS/ MINERALS	A 330mcg, Calcium 19mg, Folate 56mcg, Magnesium 9mg, Potassium 158mg			ANTIOXIDANT	Alpha Carotenoids 2mcg, Beta Carotenoids 192mcg, Lutein/Zeaxanthin 352mcg		

Source: USDA-NCC Carotenoid Database for U.S. Foods

top 20 vegetables

leaf lettuce

HEALTH BENEFIT: Excellent source of vitamin A.

SELECTION/STORAGE: Avoid lettuce with leaf edges that are slimy or dark. Leaf lettuce lasts longer if washed when brought home. Soak in a sink full of cold water, swishing it to loosen dirt. Drain, dry in a salad spinner or blot with paper towels, then refrigerate in a plastic bag for up to one week.

PREPARATION/COOKING TIPS: Rip lettuce leaves by hand. Wait until just before serving to add salad dressing.

VARIETIES: Boston, Green Leaf, Red Leaf, Romaine.

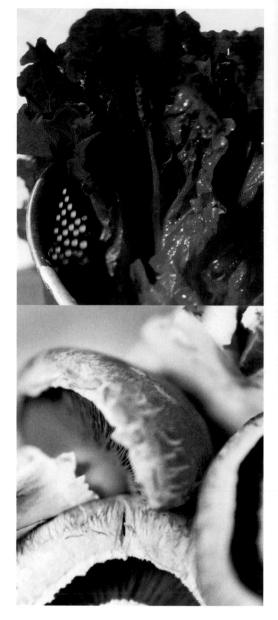

mushroom (white button)

HEALTH BENEFIT: Low-calorie, sodium-free, fat-free.

SELECTION/STORAGE: Choose mushrooms that are plump, evenly colored and have tightly closed caps. If the gills underneath are visible, the mushroom is past its prime. Store in a single layer on a tray. Cover with a damp paper towel and refrigerate for up to three days.

PREPARATION/COOKING TIPS: Never soak mushrooms. Sweep with a soft brush or take a damp paper towel and remove dirt. Trim 1/8 inch off the stems.

OTHER VARIETIES: Chanterelle, Cremini, Enoki, Hen-of-the-Woods, Morel, Oyster, Porcini, Portobello, Shiitake, White Button, Wood Ear.

NUTRITION FACTS

leaf lettuce		SERVING SIZE	CALORIES	PROTEIN	FAT	CARBOHYDRATE	DIETARY FIBER	SODIUM
	UNITED STATES	1 1/2 cups, shredded	15	1g	0g	4g	2g	30mg
	VITAMINS/ MINERALS	A 2mcg, C 18mg, Calcium 68mg, Folate 50mcg, Magnesium 11mg, Potassium 264mg			ANTIOXIDANT	Beta Carotenoids 1,272mcg, Lutein/Zeaxanthin 2,635mcg		

mushrooms		SERVING SIZE	CALORIES	PROTEIN	FAT	CARBOHYDRATE	DIETARY FIBER	SODIUM
	UNITED STATES	5 med.	20	3g	0g	3g	1g	0mg
	VITAMINS/ MINERALS	Calcium 5mg, Folate 12mcg, Magnesium 10mg, Potassium 370mg, Selenium 9mcg			ANTIOXIDANT	Alpha Carotenoids 2mcg, Beta Carotenoids 192mcg, Lutein/Zeaxanthin 352mcg		

Source: USDA-NCC Carotenoid Database for U.S. Foods

top 20 vegetables

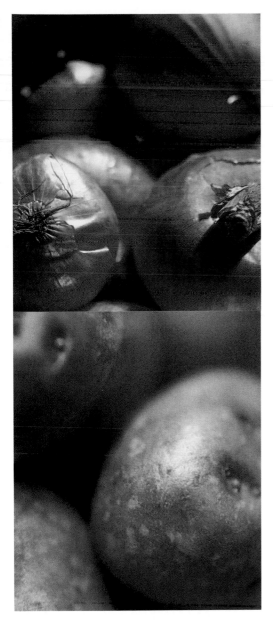

onion

HEALTH BENEFIT: High in vitamin C.

SELECTION/STORAGE: Choose firm onions that are heavy and have dry, papery skins. Avoid onions with soft spots or green sprouts. Store up to two weeks in a cool, dark, well-ventilated place, away from potatoes. Once cut, wrap tightly and refrigerate for two to three days.

PREPARATION/COOKING TIPS: Slice off root and stem ends. Remove papery skin and outer layer. Cut to desired size.

VARIETIES/BEST USES: Boiler (casseroles, soups), Dry (cooking), Knob (stir-frys), Pearl (stews), Shallots, Spanish (cooking), Sweet (sandwiches, onion rings), Vidalia® (salads, burgers, sandwiches).

potato

HEALTH BENEFIT: High in vitamin C.

SELECTION/STORAGE: Look for unblemished potatoes with no withering, cracking or sprouting of "eyes." Store for up to two weeks in a cool, dark place (50°F to 55°F).

PREPARATION/COOKING TIPS: Scrub well with a vegetable brush. Peel, if desired. Cut off any flesh that has a greenish tinge.

VARIETIES: Boiling, Fingerling, New, Red, Russet, White, Yukon Gold.

NUTRITION FACTS

onion		SERVING SIZE	CALORIES	PROTEIN	FAT	CARBOHYDRATE	DIETARY FIBER	SODIUM
	UNITED STATES	1 med.	60	1g	0g	16g	3g	5mg
	VITAMINS/ MINERALS	C 6mg, Calcium 20mg, Folate 19mcg, Magnesium 10mg, Potassium 157mg			ANTIOXIDANT	Alpha Carotenoids 6mcg, Beta Carotenoids 391mcg		

potato		SERVING SIZE	CALORIES	PROTEIN	FAT	CARBOHYDRATE	DIETARY FIBER	SODIUM
	UNITED STATES	1 med.	81	3g	0g	27g	2g	5mg
	VITAMINS/ MINERALS	C 11mg, Calcium 30mg, Folate 17mcg, Magnesium 23mg, Potassium 413mg			ANTIOXIDANT	Beta Carotenoids 6mcg		

Source: USDA-NCC Carotenoid Database for U.S. Foods

top 20 vegetables

radish

HEALTH BENEFIT: High in vitamin C.

SELECTION/STORAGE: Look for smooth, firm radishes with a minimum of surface pits. Do not buy if they have black spots, are wilted or feel spongy. Remove any leaves and refrigerate in a plastic bag for up to one week.

PREPARATION/COOKING TIPS: Wash radishes and trim roots just before using. Immerse in ice water for one hour to crisp before serving. Radishes add color and a satisfying crunch to salads.

VARIETIES: Black, Daikon, Red, White.

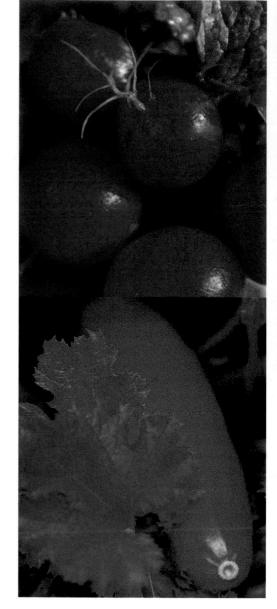

squash

HEALTH BENEFIT: High in vitamin C.

SELECTION/STORAGE: Look for yellow squash with glossy skin. Dull skin indicates that it's past its prime. The smaller the squash, the more tasty it will be. Be sure the squash is firm not spongy.

Refrigerate, unwashed, in a plastic bag for up to five days.

PREPARATION/COOKING TIPS: Do not peel before cooking. Wash, trim ends and cut to desired size. "Coins" of yellow squash are good sautéed in olive oil, and garnished with fresh basil and grated Parmesan cheese.

NUTRITION FACTS

radish		SERVING SIZE	CALORIES	PROTEIN	FAT	CARBOHYDRATE	DIETARY FIBER	SODIUM
	UNITED STATES	7 med.	15	1g	0g	3g	0g	25mg
	VITAMINS/ MINERALS	A 8mcg, C 23mg, Calcium 21mg, Folate 27mcg, Magnesium 9mg, Potassium 232mg			ANTIOXIDANT	Beta Carotenoids 1,272mcg, Lutein/Zeaxanthin 2,635mcg		

squash		SERVING SIZE	CALORIES	PROTEIN	FAT	CARBOHYDRATE	DIETARY FIBER	SODIUM
	UNITED STATES	1/2 med.	20	1g	0g	4g	2g	0mg
	VITAMINS/ MINERALS	A 338mcg, C 8mg, Calcium 21mg, Folate 23mcg, Magnesium 21mg, Potassium 212mg			ANTIOXIDANT	Beta Carotenoids 410mcg, Lutein/Zeaxanthin 2,125mcg		

Source: USDA-NCC Carotenoid Database for U.S. Foods

top 20 vegetables

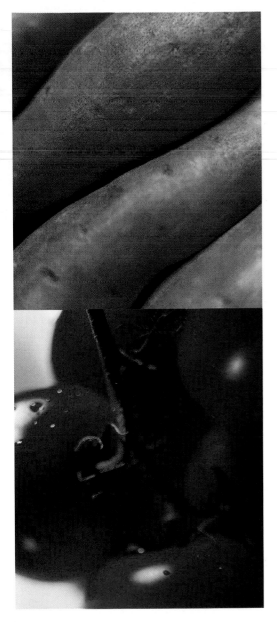

sweet potato

HEALTH BENEFIT: Excellent source of Beta-Carotene, also contains vitamin E and fiber.

SELECTION/STORAGE: Choose small to medium sweet potatoes without cracks, soft spots or blemishes. Avoid those with a greenish tinge. Do not refrigerate, but store in a cool, dark place (50⁰F to 55⁰F).

PREPARATION/COOKING TIPS: Wash well. Sweet potatoes are more nutritious if cooked in their skins and are easier to peel after they have been cooked. Prick skin with fork.

tomato

HEALTH BENEFIT: High in vitamins A and C.

SELECTION/STORAGE: Choose firm, ripe tomatoes without blemishes. Ripe tomatoes give slightly to gentle palm pressure and are fragrant and deeply colored. Store for up to two days, unrefrigerated and out of the sun.

PREPARATION/COOKING TIPS: Rinse well if eating raw. Before cooking, cut an X into the bottom of the tomato, dip tomato in boiling water for 20 seconds, plunge into cold water, then peel with fingers.

VARIETIES: Beefsteak/Vine Ripe, Cherry, Grape, Plum Roma, Slicing, Tamarillo, Teardrop, Tomatillo.

NUTRITION FACTS

sweet potato

	SERVING SIZE	CALORIES	PROTEIN	FAT	CARBOHYDRATE	DIETARY FIBER	SODIUM
UNITED STATES	1 med.	136	2g	0g	33g	4g	17mg
VITAMINS/MINERALS	A 20,063mcg, C 23mg, Potassium 204mg			ANTIOXIDANT	Beta Carotenoids 9,180mcg		

tomato

	SERVING SIZE	CALORIES	PROTEIN	FAT	CARBOHYDRATE	DIETARY FIBER	SODIUM
UNITED STATES	1 med.	35	1g	0.5g	7g	1g	0mg
VITAMINS/MINERALS	A 623mcg, C 10mg, Calcium 5mg, Folate 15mcg, Magnesium 11mg, Potassium 222mg			ANTIOXIDANT	Alpha Carotenoids 112mcg, Beta Carotenoids 393mcg, Lutein/Zeaxanthin 130mcg, Lycopene 3,025mcg		

Source: USDA-NCC Carotenoid Database for U.S. Foods

herbs

	DESCRIPTION	TASTE	SELECTION
arugula	Features leaves with slightly jagged edges.	Distinct, peppery bite.	Look for emerald-green leaves 2 to 4 inches long.
basil	Bright green, glossy leaves.	Pungent; a cross between licorice and cloves.	Choose leaves that are fresh, unspotted and fragrant.
bay leaf	Smooth, tough, glossy, bright green leaves.	Aromatic and pungent.	Select leaves free from discoloration.
chervil	A member of the carrot family.	Reminiscent of licorice, anise or tarragon.	Looks like parsley. Look for feathery, delicate green leaves with heady aroma.
chives	Delicate, hollow green blades.	Like a mild onion.	Choose chives with a uniform (Garlic Chives: flat blades) (Garlic Chives: midly garlic) green color.
cilantro	Leaves resemble parsley.	Pungent, distinctive and strong.	Look for fresh, leafy bunches with roots still attached.
cinnamon	Quills, sticks or powdered.	Spicy, nutty sweet.	Ceylon cinnamon is less sweet. Cassia cinnamon is more common.
dill	Feathery, fern-like leaves.	Aromatic.	Select deep-green crisp-looking leaves.
fennel	Bulb, stalks and flowery greens.	Sweeter, more delicate than anise.	Choose clean, crisp, pearly bulbs without browning or cracks.
garlic	White bulb. Pungent.	Nutty, sweet when roasted.	Pick firm heads without green growth.
gingerroot	Beige, knobby root.	Spicy, fragrant and pungent.	Look for robust roots without withering or cracking.
horseradish root	Spiky green leaves, large brown root.	Pungent.	Look for firm roots without bruises.
italian parsley	Flat pointed leaves, resembles cilantro.	Stronger than curly-leafed parsley	Select fresh leaves with no sign of wilting.

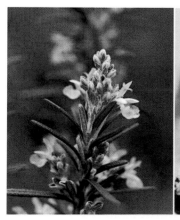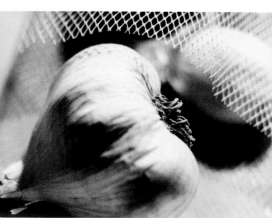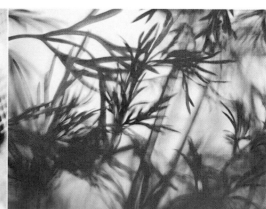

STORAGE	PREPARATION	COOKING TIPS
Wrap roots in damp paper towel; refrigerate up to 2 days.	Wash thoroughly. Chop off roots and thick stems.	Add to salad greens and pasta.
Wrap in damp paper towels and refrigerate in plastic bag.	Wash and remove leaves from main stems.	Try in pasta sauce, in salads or on bruschetta. Source of iron, used as a cold remedy.
Store in a plastic bag in the refrigerator up to 3 days.	Rinse and towel dry.	Add to stews, soups, vegetables and meat dishes for aroma and flavor. Remove bay leaves before serving.
Store in plastic bag in the refrigerator for 2 days.	Rinse and towel dry. Chop finely.	Add to soups, stews, vegetables, meat or fish dishes just before serving. Use as garnish.
Store in a plastic bag in the refrigerator up to 1 week.	Rinse and towel dry. Snip with scissors to desired length.	Use as garnish. Add to dish at the last moment. Complements potatoes, carrots and green beans.
Place roots in glass of water. Refrigerate. Loosely cover leaves with plastic wrap.	Rinse when ready for use. Cut off roots and thick stems. Spin dry. Chop.	Fresh leaves are used in Mexican, Mediterranean and Chinese dishes. Use in salsa, guacamole, soups, salads, stews or stir-frys.
Keep in airtight container in a cool, dark place.	Remove cinnamon sticks before serving.	Use in warm winter drinks or flavored iced tea. Flavor chutney, stews and pickled foods.
Refrigerate, wrapped, for a few days.	Chop off thick stems and mince dill with scissors.	Great in potato and egg salads and with fish. Add near the end of cooking time.
Wrap tightly in plastic and refrigerate up to 4 days.	Slice off the tough bottom of the bulb. Peel off layers and discard hard core. If using stalks, peel first.	Cut or slice as desired to use raw in salads. Braise, boil, saute, bake, broil or grill.
Store in cool, dark bin.	Remove cloves from head. Press with flat of knife to loosen skin.	To roast, do not peel first. Drizzle with olive oil and seal tightly in foil. Bake for 45 minutes. Spread tender cloves on crusty bread or add to mashed potatoes.
Store in the refrigerator for up to 3 weeks. Slice unpeeled ginger and place in a jar with sherry. Refrigerate up to 3 months.	Peel the thin beige skin away. Mince for more flavor.	Use half the amount of fresh gingerroot in recipes calling for dried. Use in stir-fried and curry dishes.
Grate and keep in bottle of salted vinegar. Cut root in chunks and freeze.	Peel away brown skin and cut away hard inner portion. Grate.	Use on roast beef or add to seafood cocktail sauce.
Place in glass of water, cover with plastic bag and refrigerate.	Remove thick stems and chop leaves to desired size.	Used to balance garlic dishes and as a garnish.

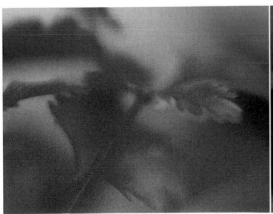 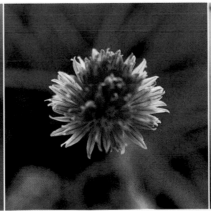 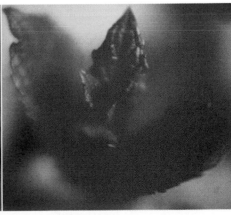

herbs

	DESCRIPTION	TASTE	SELECTION
lemongrass	Pale yellow-green stalks with bulbous bases.	Pungent citrus taste, similar to lime zest.	The greener the stalk, the fresher it is.
marjoram	Pale green, oval 1/2 to inch-long leaves.	Resembles sweet oregano.	Select marjoram that appears fresh and unwilted.
mint	Bright-green leaves with purplish stems.	Has a cool and refreshing bite.	Choose fresh mint with evenly colored leaves.
oregano	Small, round, green leaves.	Strong and spicy.	Look for fresh leaves with no brown spots.
parsley	Curly leaves.	A natural breath freshener.	Choose parsley with bright-green, curly leaves.
parsley root	Creamy white skin, resembles a small parsnip.	Tastes like a combination of carrots and celery.	Select parsley roots with the fresh, unwilted greens attached, creamy white and unblemished roots.
rhubarb	Pink to cherry-red stalks.	Tart.	Choose firm stalks that are fresh and crisp.
rosemary	Silvery green, spiky leaves.	A combination of lemon and pine.	Look for fresh, velvety sprigs that show no signs of drying out.
sage	Narrow, oval gray-green leaves.	Earthy mint.	Look for soft, silvery green leaves with no brown spots.
savory	Resembles thyme, but with larger leaves.	Similar to thyme, but more bitter.	Look for fresh leaves that are shiny on the upper surface with no brown spots.
sorrel	Pale to dark-green spinach-shaped leaves.	Lemony flavor.	Look for bunches with firm, green leaves and stems with no spots or signs of wilting.
tarragon	Deep-green sprigs with long, narrow, pointed leaves.	Peppery with anise overtones.	Look for deep-green tarragon sprigs with long, narrow, pointed leaves.
thyme	Gray-green leaves.	Sharp, peppery taste.	Look for fragrant, fresh-looking leaves.

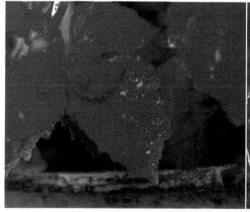
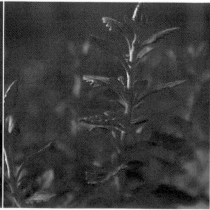
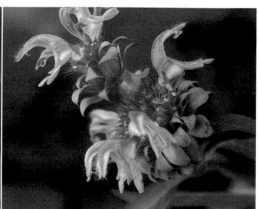

STORAGE	PREPARATION	COOKING TIPS
Wrap each stalk in foil and refrigerate for up to 2 weeks.	Pound then discard outer leaves with a mallet to release fragrant oils.	Outer leaves are inedible. Use in Thai dishes.
Wrap leaves in damp paper towels, place in plastic bag and refrigerate.	Snip rinsed leaves from the stem; chop.	Add to salads, eggs, butter sauces, dressing, soups, beans or pasta.
Refrigerate in glass of water, stems down, covered with plastic bag.	Wash, dry and snip off leaves. Use whole or chopped.	Use with peas, carrots, new potatoes, tea, lamb or fruit salad. Freshens breath, aids digestion.
Refrigerate in a plastic bag.	Wash and pat dry. Snip leaves from stems and chop.	Add to pasta, dressings, sauces, poultry, seafood or any tomato dish, source of iron. Aids in memory, anti-yeast activity.
Wrap in paper towels and refrigerate in a plastic bag for up to 1 week.	Revive by cutting off one inch of stem, placing in cold water and refrigerating for 1 hour. Chop or snip.	Flavor soups or sauces or use as garnish. vitamin A rich.
Refrigerate in a plastic bag for up to 1 week.	Trim greens. Scrub and peel roots.	Purée, cream or steam. Add to mashed potatoes (1 part parsley roots/3 parts potatoes).
Refrigerate, unwashed, in a plastic bag for 1 week.	Remove any fibrous strings and leaves.	Never eat the leaves. Stew, bake in pies, or preserve in jelly.
Refrigerate in a plastic bag for up to 1 week.	Rinse, pat dry and chop to desired size.	Use whole sprigs in soups or stews (remove before serving), in cavities of chicken or with fish. Use in moderation. Add to tea to soothe headaches.
Refrigerate, unwashed, in a paper towel for up to 4 days.	Chop, snip or use leaves whole.	Great with pork, polenta, poultry and in stuffing. A digestive aid, relieves painful gums.
Refrigerate in a plastic bag for 3 or 4 days.	Rinse sprigs, dry with paper towels then snip leaves from stem.	Chop leaves or use whole with beans, pork, poultry, veal or cabbage.
Refrigerate, unwashed, in plastic bag for up to 2 days.	Wash and drain thoroughly then remove leaves from stems.	Use as salad greens, in soups or stews.
Wrap and refrigerate for up to 2 days.	Wash sprigs, dry with paper towels and remove thick stems.	Use caution when seasoning with this assertive herb as it can easily overwhelm other ingredients.
Wrap in barely damp paper towel and refrigerate in plastic bag for up to 5 days.	Wash, towel dry and snip with kitchen scissors.	Use sparingly to flavor soups and gravies, and in tomato, onion and corn dishes. Source of iron. As a tea, quiets irritable bowel.

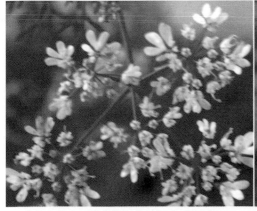
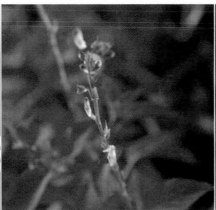
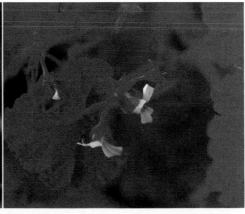

wake up to a
healthy start

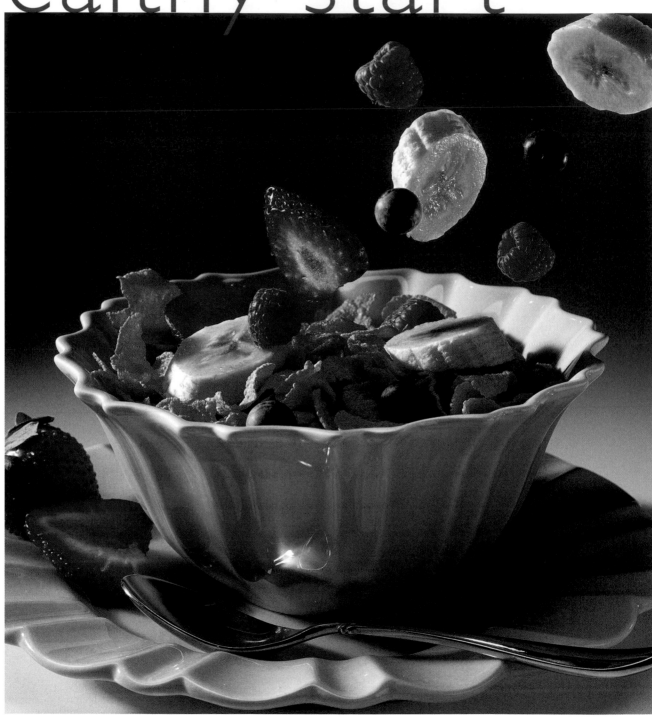

Get a jump on five servings of fruit and vegetables for the day by building your breakfasts and brunches around these eye-opening recipes.

fruitful beginnings

FRESH FRUIT IS ONE OF LIFE'S sweet pleasures. From crisp apples to luscious berries or juicy peaches, there's nothing like fruit to perk up meals—especially since it's generally low in calories and high in vitamins and fiber. What's more, eating fresh fruit for breakfast is a great way to meet your 5 A Day goal.

Now, it's easier than ever to eat a variety of fruit because many—including grapes, peaches, nectarines, plums, raspberries, blueberries, blackberries, pears, apples and kiwifruit—are available year-round. The fruit you purchase "in season" are from the many fruit-growing areas in the United States. The ones you purchase "out of season" are imported from other parts of the world, like Chile.

To help you enjoy fresh fruit at its best, here are some tips for selecting, ripening, storing and serving fresh fruit.

SELECTING: Choose well-shaped fruit that has good color for its variety. Berries and grapes should be plump and juicy. Stone fruit, such as peaches, nectarines and plums, should be slightly firm. Purchase pears when firm, then ripen at home until they yield to gentle pressure. Apples should be firm and crisp.

RIPENING: If unripe when purchased, nectarines, peaches, plums and pears can be ripened at home in a closed paper bag at room temperature for several days. Add an apple or ripe banana to speed up the ripening.

STORING: Don't wash fruit until just before serving. The bloom—the dusty coating that appears on some fruit—helps keep them fresh. Once ripe, keep tree fruit and grapes in a plastic bag in the refrigerator. Store berries tightly wrapped in their original packaging (or in a single layer in a tightly covered container) in the refrigerator until you are ready to use them.

SERVING: For best flavor, serve fruit at room temperature.

6 ways to enjoy fruit

1 BAKE A BATCH OF LOW-FAT MUFFINS USING whatever fruit is in season.

2 FOR A HEARTY AND HEALTHY BREAKFAST, ENJOY low-fat granola mixed with fat-free yogurt and mixed fruit.

3 TOP WAFFLES OR PANCAKES WITH BLUEBERRIES, blackberries, raspberries or sliced peaches or nectarines, and fat-free sour cream.

4 AS PART OF A BREAKFAST ON THE GO, NIBBLE ON frozen blueberries or grapes.

5 FOR A BRUNCH BEVERAGE, IN A BLENDER CONTAINER, combine 1 peeled peach or nectarine, cut into chunks; 1/2 cup milk; 1/2 cup orange juice; 1 tablespoon honey; 1/4 teaspoon almond extract; and 2 ice cubes, cracked. Cover and blend until smooth.

6 SPREAD TOASTED ENGLISH MUFFINS OR BAGELS WITH fat-free cream cheese and top with sliced kiwifruit, halved grapes, blueberries, raspberries or blackberries.

breakfast
healthy recipes

BRUNCH FRUIT COMPOTE

EASY RECIPE:

2 cups water

1 cup fresh mint leaves

1/3 cup honey

1 can (6-oz.) frozen
lemonade concentrate

10 cups assorted fresh fruit (such as
blueberries, blackberries, halved
kiwifruit slices, halved cherries,
sliced plums, fresh pineapple
chunks, halved strawberries, sliced
peaches, orange sections, halved
seedless grapes and cantaloupe
and/or watermelon balls)

Fresh mint sprigs (optional)

EASY STEPS:

In a medium saucepan, combine
water, mint, and honey. Bring
mixture to a boil. Reduce heat and
simmer, covered, for 10 minutes.
Strain into a medium mixing
bowl, discarding the mint. Stir in
lemonade concentrate. Cover, if
desired; chill for up to 24 hours.

Place the fruit in a large serving
bowl. Pour the lemonade mixture
over fruit. Cover and chill until
needed, up to 8 hours. (If toting,
transfer to a storage container and
keep on ice in a cooler until
serving time.) Toss before serving.
Garnish each serving with a mint
sprig, if desired.

Makes 10 to 12 servings.

Nutrition facts per serving: 153 calories
(4% from fat), 1 g total fat (0 g saturated fat),
0 mg cholesterol, 10 mg sodium,
39 g carbohydrate, 4 g dietary fiber,
1 g protein.

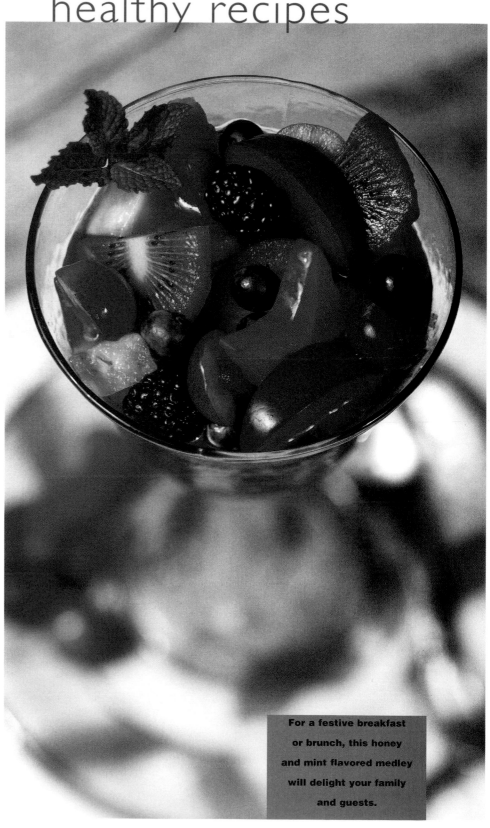

For a festive breakfast
or brunch, this honey
and mint flavored medley
will delight your family
and guests.

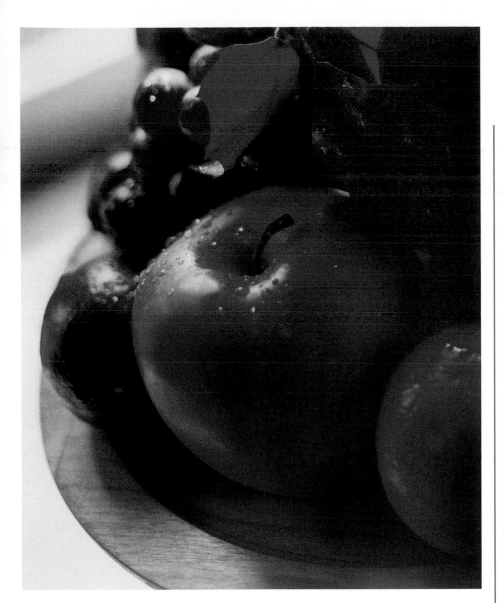

GOLDEN APPLE OATMEAL

Dining alone? Jazz up your morning with this oatmeal, apple, and spice combo that's easy to make.

EASY RECIPE:

1 cup chopped Golden Delicious apple

2/3 cup apple juice

2/3 cup water

1/8 tsp. salt (optional)

Dash ground cinnamon

Dash ground nutmeg

2/3 cup quick-cooking rolled oats, uncooked

EASY STEPS:

In a small saucepan, combine the apple, apple juice, water, salt (if desired), cinnamon and nutmeg; bring to a boil. Stir in the rolled oats; cook for 1 minute. Remove from heat. Cover and let stand for several minutes before serving.
Makes 2 servings.

Nutrition facts per serving: 176 calories (10% from fat), 2 g total fat (0 g saturated fat), 0 mg cholesterol, 6 mg sodium, 36 g carbohydrate, 4 g dietary fiber, 4 g protein.

MICROWAVE BREAKFAST COBBLER

For a cozy taste of home, try this warm, sweet breakfast treat.

EASY RECIPE:

3 (16-oz.) peaches, sliced

3 (16-oz.) pears, halved

1 cup halved, pitted prunes (about 6 oz.)

1 tsp. grated orange peel

1/3 cup fresh orange juice

1½ cups reduced-fat granola

Plain low-fat yogurt (optional)

EASY STEPS:

In a shallow 6-cup microwave-safe bowl, toss together the peaches, pears, prunes, orange peel and orange juice. Top with granola. Microwave on 100% power (high) about 5 minutes or until heated through. Let stand for 2 minutes. Spoon into bowls. Serve with plain yogurt, if desired.
Makes 4 to 6 servings.

Nutrition facts per serving: 319 calories (7% from fat), 3 g total fat (0 g saturated fat), 0 mg cholesterol, 50 mg sodium, 76 g carbohydrate, 10 g dietary fiber, 4 g protein.

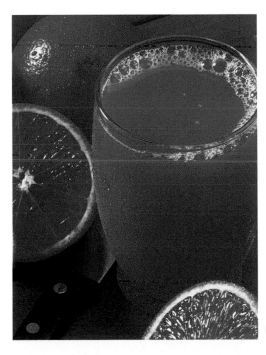

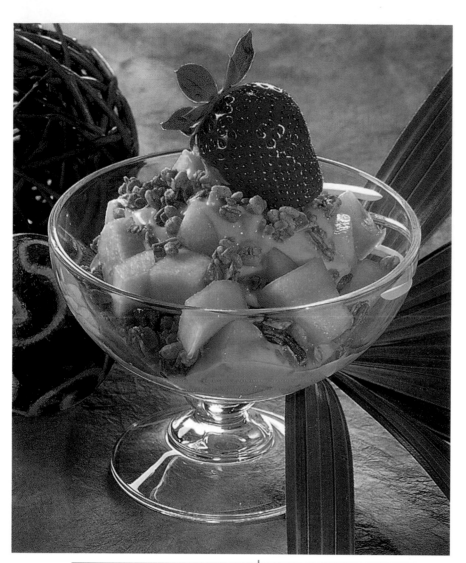

MELON CRUNCH PARFAIT

Creamy, crunchy and just sweet enough, this layered treat is a great breakfast option.

EASY RECIPE:

1 medium honeydew melon

1 cup low-fat vanilla yogurt

1 tbsp. brown sugar

1 cup low-fat granola

4 strawberries

EASY STEPS:

Cut honeydew into grape-size cubes. Combine yogurt and brown sugar. Spoon half the yogurt mixture into 4 dessert glasses. Top with half of the melon cubes. Add half the granola. Repeat. Garnish with strawberries. Makes 4 servings.

Nutrition facts per serving: 270 calories (9% from fat), 3 g total fat, 3 mg cholesterol, 70 mg sodium, 62 g carbohydrate, 6 g protein.

CITRUS STAR CUPS

EASY RECIPE:

2 grapefruit

2 oranges, peeled and cut into bite-size pieces

1 tangerine, peeled and sectioned

1/2 lb. red seedless grapes

1/4 cup shredded coconut

EASY STEPS:

Make sawtooth cuts all around grapefruit. Twist and pull grapefruit apart. Scoop out pulp and cut it into bite-size pieces. Set grapefruit "shells" aside. Toss all fruit in a bowl with coconut. Spoon fruit in the grapefruit shells.
Makes 4 servings.

Nutrition facts per serving: 134 calories, 1 g total fat, 0 mg cholesterol, 5 mg sodium, 33 g carbohydrate, 4 g dietary fiber, 2 g protein.

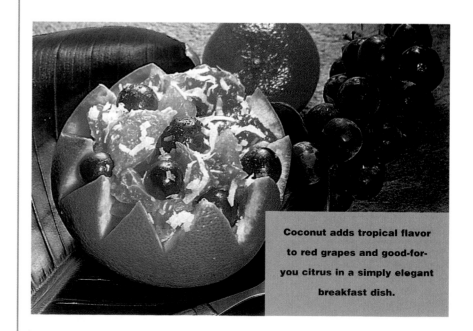

Coconut adds tropical flavor to red grapes and good-for-you citrus in a simply elegant breakfast dish.

TROPICAL FRUIT SALAD

Serve this yogurt and fresh fruit medley with spicy Mexican or Caribbean entrées. For the best flavor, be sure to use ripe mangoes—ones that yield to gentle pressure and have a fruity aroma.

EASY RECIPE:

1 cup cubed mango

1 large banana, sliced

1 cup cubed fresh pineapple

1 cup cubed avocado

1 cup chopped orange

1/2 cup plain nonfat yogurt

3 tbsp. sugar

2 tbsp. orange juice

1/4 cup shredded coconut (optional)

EASY STEPS:

In a medium bowl, combine mango, banana, pineapple, avocado and orange. Stir together yogurt, sugar and orange juice; spoon over fruit and mix well. Cover and chill for 30 minutes. Sprinkle with shredded coconut before serving, if desired. Makes 4 servings.

Nutrition facts per serving: 360 calories (28% from fat), 11 g total fat, 2 mg cholesterol, 230 mg sodium, 63 g carbohydrate, 7 g dietary fiber, 10 g protein.

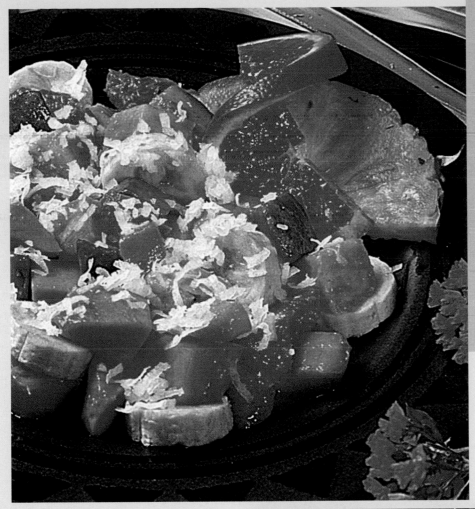

GRAPEFRUIT SUNRISER

EASY RECIPE:

1½ cups freshly juiced red grapefruit (about 2 grapefruit)

8 large strawberries (fresh or frozen)

2 medium bananas

1 carton (8 oz.) strawberry-banana yogurt

2 tbsp. honey

1 cup crushed ice

EASY STEPS:

Pour juice into a blender and add strawberries. Cut bananas into chunks. Add bananas and all other ingredients to blender and blend until smooth. Makes 4 (8-oz.) servings.

Nutrition facts per serving: 60 calories (0% from fat), 0 g total fat, 0 mg cholesterol, 0 mg sodium, 16 g carbohydrate, 6 g dietary fiber, 1 g protein.

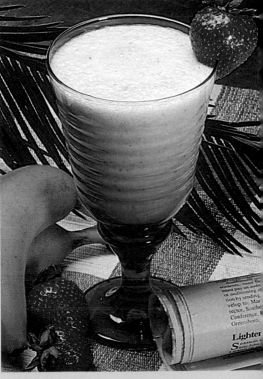

This tangy and sweet breakfast drink is packed with vitamin C...the perfect way to start any day.

out-of-the slump
lunches

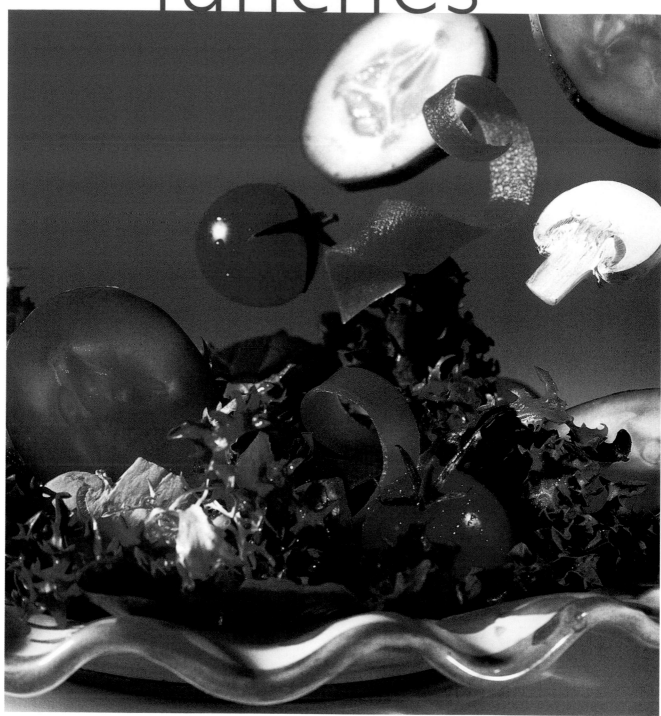

Take a little time at noon to enjoy one of these bountiful dishes and you'll be renewed for an afternoon of work or play.

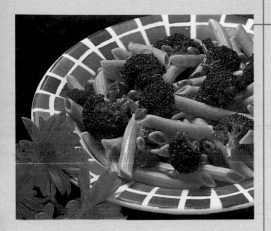

BROCCOLI PASTA WITH PINE NUTS

Pignoli, also known as pine nuts, make a crunchy garnish for this broccoli and pasta toss.

EASY RECIPE:

1 head broccoli, trimmed
1 lb. penne pasta, cooked and drained
1 red bell pepper, seeded and chopped
1/2 cup orange juice
1/4 cup red wine vinegar
2 tbsp. olive oil
1/4 cup pine nuts, toasted
Orange twists (optional)

EASY STEPS:

Cut broccoli into florets and the stems into 1/2-inch disks. Place a steamer basket in a large saucepan and add water to just below the steamer basket. Bring to a boil. Add broccoli; cover and reduce heat. After 4 minutes, check broccoli with a fork. (The fork should easily pierce the stalk.) Remove from heat. In a large bowl toss together broccoli, pasta and bell pepper. In a small bowl whisk together orange juice, vinegar and olive oil. Pour mixture over pasta mixture, tossing to coat. Sprinkle with pine nuts. Garnish each serving with an orange twist, if desired.
Makes 4 servings.

Nutrition facts per serving: 379 calories (21% from fat), 9 g total fat, 0 mg cholesterol, 12 mg sodium, 62 g carbohydrate, 3 g dietary fiber, 12 g protein.

CHICKEN CITRUS SALAD

EASY RECIPE:

Citrus Vinaigrette
2 tbsp. fresh orange juice
2 tbsp. red wine vinegar
2 tsp. olive oil
2 tsp. honey
1¼ tsp. purchased
    Dijon-style mustard
Salad
4 small skinless, boneless chicken breast halves (12 oz. total)
4 cups torn mixed salad greens
2 medium oranges, peeled and sectioned
Fresh strawberries (optional)

EASY STEPS:

To make the vinaigrette: In a small bowl combine orange juice, vinegar, oil, honey and mustard. Set aside.

To make the salad: Place chicken on a grill rack over medium-hot coals. Grill, uncovered, for 6 minutes. Turn the chicken; grill for 6 to 9 minutes more or until the chicken is tender and no longer pink. Cut into 1/2-inch-thick slices.

In a large bowl toss mixed greens and oranges. Arrange the greens mixture on 4 salad plates. Place a sliced chicken breast on each plate. Drizzle with vinaigrette. Garnish with strawberries, if desired.
Makes 4 servings.

Nutrition facts per serving: 150 calories (30% from fat), 5 g total fat (1 g saturated fat), 45 mg cholesterol, 85 mg sodium, 9 g carbohydrate, 1 g dietary fiber, 17 g protein.

Made with chicken and refreshing sweet oranges—this salad is delightfully low in fat.

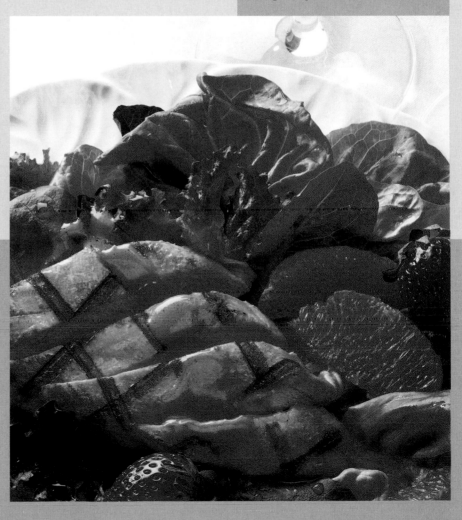

RIVIERA SALAD

EASY RECIPE:

6 medium potatoes (about 2 pounds), quartered and cooked

2/3 cup prepared low-calorie Italian salad dressing

Lettuce leaves

3 cups fresh vegetables (such as asparagus, green beans and/or snow peas), steamed, drained and cooled

2 medium tomatoes, sliced

2 (6½-oz.) cans low-sodium chunk light tuna (water pack), drained and flaked

1 cup sliced fresh mushrooms

1 bunch radishes, trimmed

Fresh parsley sprigs

EASY STEPS:

In large bowl toss potatoes with half of the salad dressing. Cover; chill. Line 2 medium platters with lettuce. Arrange potatoes and remaining ingredients on platters. Serve with the remaining dressing.
Makes 6 servings.

Nutrition facts per serving: 270 calories (14% from fat), 4 g total fat (0 g saturated fat), 2 mg cholesterol, 358 mg sodium, 42 g carbohydrate, 4 g dietary fiber, 18 g protein.

A main course salad that's both filling and light, the Riviera Salad makes a great lunch selection.

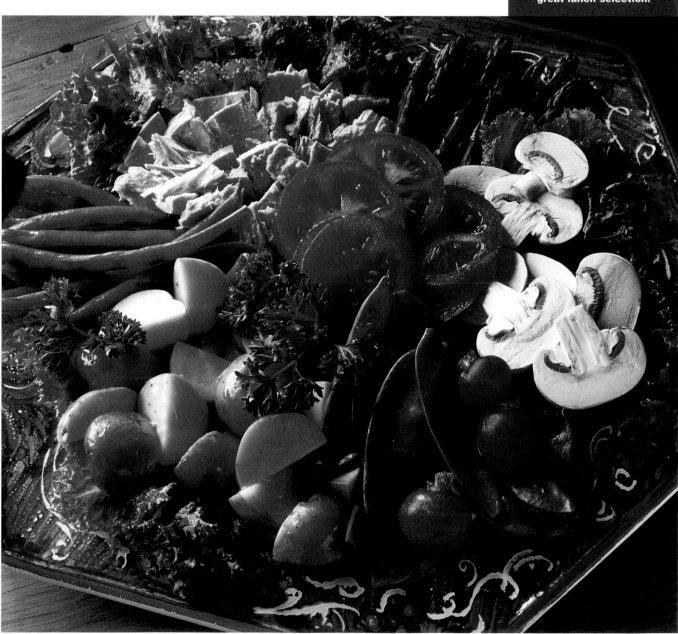

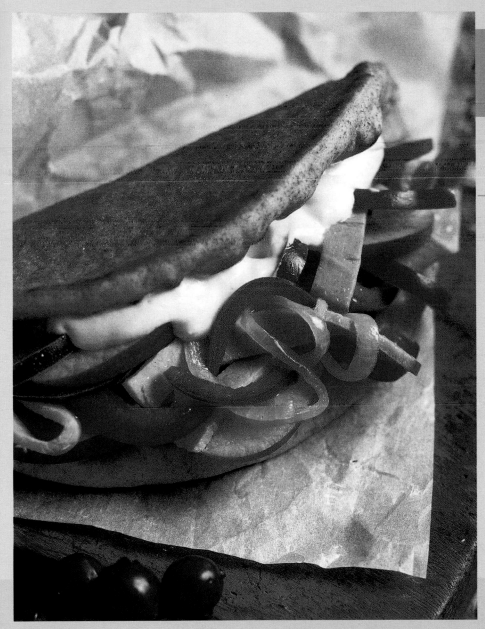

To quickly cut and core the apple, just quarter it, cut the core from each section and slice each quarter.

SUNSHINE SPINACH SALAD

This flavorful blend of greens, fruit and crisp vegetables is filling and nutritious midday fare.

EASY RECIPE:

5 cups torn fresh spinach

2 medium oranges, peeled and cut into bite-size pieces

1 medium cucumber, sliced

1/2 medium red onion, thinly sliced

1/2 medium red sweet pepper, sliced

1/3 cup purchased fat-free Italian salad dressing

EASY STEPS:

In a large bowl toss together spinach, oranges, cucumber, onion and red pepper. Add salad dressing and toss again. Serve immediately. Makes 5 servings.

Nutrition facts per serving: 41 calories (6% from fat), 0 g total fat (0 g saturated fat), 0 mg cholesterol, 268 mg sodium, 8 g carbohydrate, 2 g dietary fiber, 2 g protein.

APPLE-TURKEY GYROS

EASY RECIPE:

1 medium Winesap or Golden Delicious apple, cored and thinly-sliced

2 tbsp. fresh lemon juice

1 cup thinly-sliced onion

1 medium red sweet pepper, cut into thin strips

1 medium green pepper, cut into thin strips

1 tbsp. cooking oil

8 oz. cooked turkey breast, cut into thin strips

6 pita bread rounds, lightly toasted

1/2 cup plain low-fat yogurt

EASY STEPS:

Toss apple with lemon juice; set aside. In a large nonstick skillet cook and stir onion, red pepper and green pepper in hot oil until crisp-tender. Stir in turkey; cook and stir until heated through. Stir in apple mixture.

Fold the pita rounds in half and fill with the turkey mixture; drizzle with the yogurt. Serve warm. Makes 6 servings.

Nutrition facts per serving: 279 calories (15% from fat), 5 g total fat (1 g saturated fat), 27 mg cholesterol, 360 mg sodium, 41 g carbohydrate, 1 g dietary fiber, 18 g protein.

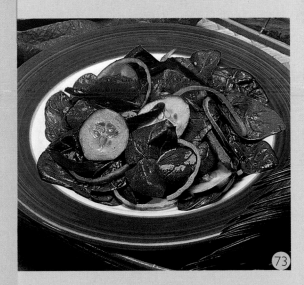

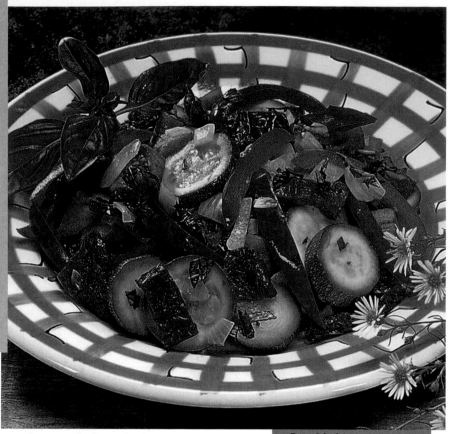

GRILLED PORTOBELLO SANDWICH

EASY RECIPE:

6 portobello mushrooms

3 bell peppers

5 cloves garlic, minced

1/2 cup balsamic vinegar

2 tsp. olive oil

1 tsp. chopped fresh basil

1 tsp. chopped fresh parsley (optional)

6 kaiser rolls, split

Lettuce or arugula leaves (optional)

EASY STEPS:

Discard portobello stems and wipe mushrooms with a damp paper towel. Quarter peppers. Whisk together vinegar, oil, herbs, and garlic; season with salt and pepper. Coat peppers and mushrooms with mixture in two separate containers; marinate for 1 hour. Preheat grill. Spray grill rack with nonstick cooking spray. Grill mushrooms and peppers 3 to 4 minutes per side over medium heat or until tender. Thinly slice mushrooms. Toast roll halves on grill. Fill rolls with mushrooms and peppers. Add lettuce leaves or arugula, if desired. Makes 6 servings.

Nutrition facts per serving: 164 calories (21% from fat), 4 g total fat, 0 mg cholesterol, 243 mg sodium, 28 g carbohydrate, 1 g dietary fiber, 5 g protein.

SUN-DRIED TOMATO RATATOUILLE

EASY RECIPE:

1 medium eggplant, peeled and diced

1 cup sun-dried tomatoes (not oil pack)

2 medium zucchini, sliced

2 red or green bell peppers, sliced

3 yellow onions, peeled and diced

6 garlic cloves, chopped

1 cup chicken broth

3 sprigs fresh basil, chopped

EASY STEPS:

Place eggplant cubes in a large bowl of water. Use kitchen scissors to cut tomatoes in half. Drain eggplant. Cook zucchini, peppers, tomatoes, onions and garlic in chicken broth 3 to 4 minutes or until peppers are tender. Season to taste with salt and pepper. Top vegetables with fresh basil. Makes 4 servings.

Nutrition facts per serving: 137 calories (8% from fat), 1 g total fat, less than 300 mg cholesterol, 402 mg sodium, 30 g carbohydrate, 9 g dietary fiber, 6 g protein.

Sun-dried tomatoes can be used as colorful, edible garnishes or as a great addition to dishes for flavor.

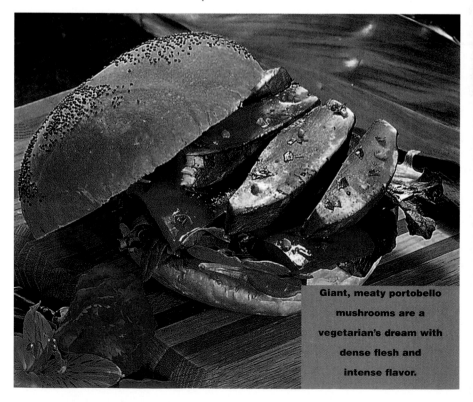

Giant, meaty portobello mushrooms are a vegetarian's dream with dense flesh and intense flavor.

midday delights

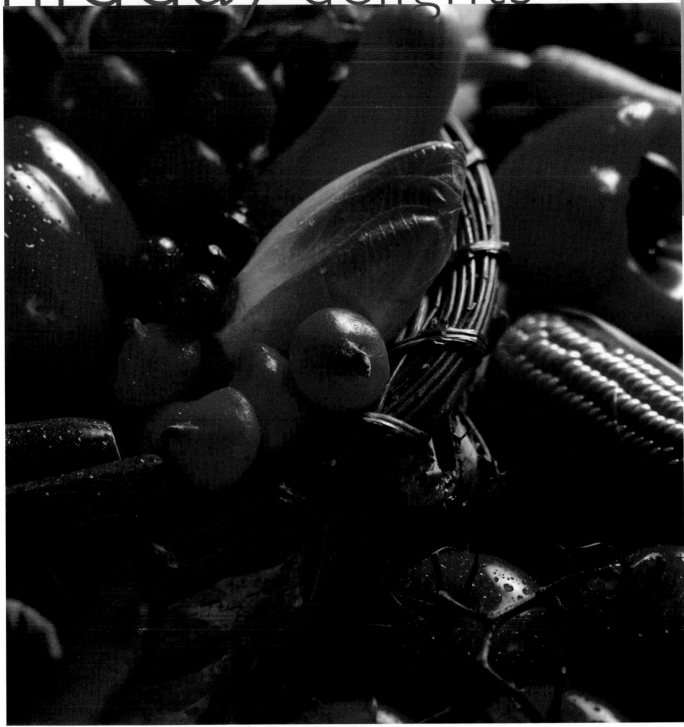

When between-meal hunger hits, dig in!
These snacks will make your day—and help you achieve your 5 A Day goal.

STRAWBERRY-YOGURT SHAKE

Here's a fruity drink you'll enjoy sipping on a hot summer day. It's not only refreshing, it also supplies you with one full serving of fruit.

EASY RECIPE:

1/2 cup unsweetened pineapple juice

3/4 cup plain low-fat yogurt

1½ cups frozen unsweetened whole strawberries

1 tsp. sugar

2 fresh strawberry fans (optional)

EASY STEPS:

Pour juice in blender container. Add yogurt, frozen strawberries and sugar. Cover and blend until smooth. Pour into 2 tall glasses. Garnish each glass with a strawberry fan, if desired.

Makes 2 (12-oz.) servings.

Nutrition facts per serving: 131 calories (12% from fat), 2 g total fat (1 g saturated fat), 5 mg cholesterol, 61 mg sodium, 25 g carbohydrate, 2 g dietary fiber, 5 g protein.

WATERMELON SMOOTHIE

Turn this creamy watermelon sipper into a different fruit drink by replacing the watermelon with 2 cups of cantaloupe or honeydew chunks or peach slices.

EASY RECIPE:

2 cups seeded watermelon chunks

1 cup cracked ice

1/2 cup plain low-fat yogurt

1 tablespoon sugar

1/2 teaspoon ground ginger

1/8 teaspoon almond extract

Watermelon balls (optional)

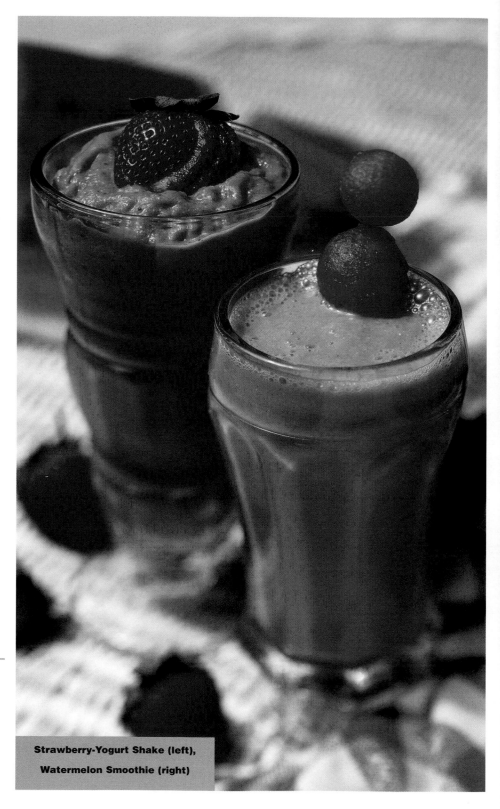

Strawberry-Yogurt Shake (left), Watermelon Smoothie (right)

In a blender container, combine the 2 cups watermelon, ice, yogurt, sugar, ginger and almond extract. Cover and blend until smooth. Pour into 2 tall glasses. If desired, garnish each serving with watermelon balls. Makes 2 (8-oz.) servings.

Nutrition facts per serving: 114 calories (12% from fat), 2 g total fat (1 g saturated fat), 4 mg cholesterol, 44 mg sodium, 22 g carbohydrate, 1 g dietary fiber, 4 g protein.

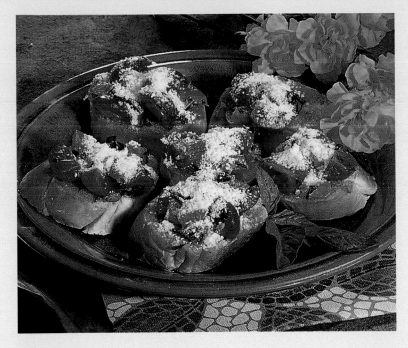

GRILLED BRUSCHETTA TOASTS

For flavorful bruschetta, choose red cherry or grape tomatoes.

EASY RECIPE:

1 loaf Italian bread, cut in 1-inch slices

1 cup cherry tomatoes, quartered

1 small yellow bell peppers, chopped

2 tbsp. olive oil

2 tbsp. chopped fresh basil

1 clove garlic, minced

3 tbsp. grated Parmesan cheese

EASY STEPS:

Preheat grill. Brush bread with 1 tablespoon olive oil. Lightly toast both sides of bread slices about 2 minutes per side. Combine tomatoes, pepper, 1 tablespoon oil, basil and garlic. Spoon tomato mixture onto toast and sprinkle with cheese. Makes 8 servings.

Nutrition facts per serving: 116 calories (26% from fat), 3 g total fat, 1 mg cholesterol, 213 mg sodium, 18 g carbohydrate, 1 g dietary fiber, 4 g protein.

MELON SPICY DIP

EASY RECIPE:

1 cup low-fat cottage cheese

2 tbsp. honey

1/2 tsp. ground cinnamon

1/4 tsp. ground nutmeg

2 medium melons such as cantaloupe and honeydew, cubed

EASY STEPS:

Place cottage cheese, honey, cinnamon and nutmeg in a blender container or food processor. Blend until smooth. Serve with melon cubes.
Makes 4 servings.

Nutrition facts per serving: 246 calories (9% from fat), 2 g total fat, 5 mg cholesterol, 27 mg sodium, 50 g carbohydrate, 4 g dietary fiber, 12 g protein.

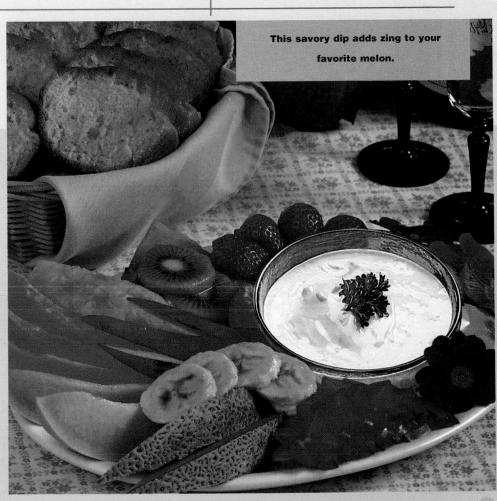

This savory dip adds zing to your favorite melon.

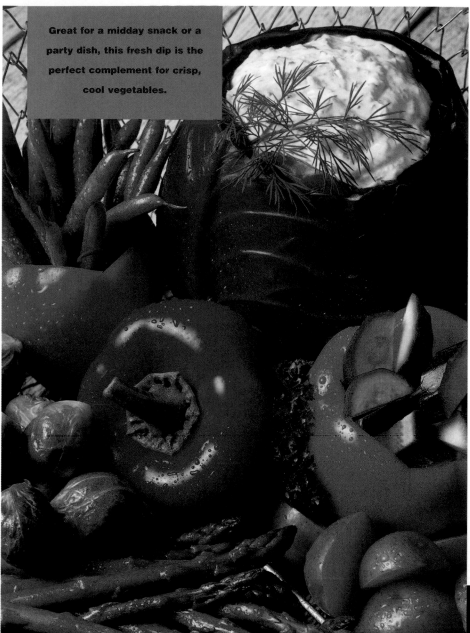

Great for a midday snack or a party dish, this fresh dip is the perfect complement for crisp, cool vegetables.

FROZEN PINEAPPLE BARS

This frozen treat couldn't be easier to make! Delicious with pineapple, try these bars with any summer fruit, such as strawberries, oranges or peaches.

EASY RECIPE:

2 cups fresh peeled and cubed pineapple

1 tsp. lemon juice

1 tbsp. sugar (optional)

EASY STEPS:

Place the fruit in a blender container. Cover and blend until smooth, adding 1 to 2 tablespoons water, if necessary. Add lemon juice and sugar, if desired. Cover and blend until well mixed. Pour into 4-ounce ice-pop molds or paper cups; insert sticks. Freeze until solid. Makes 4 bars.

Nutrition facts per serving: 23 calories (10% from fat), 0 g total fat (0 g saturated fat), 0 mg cholesterol, 1 mg sodium, 5 g carbohydrate, 1 g dietary fiber, 0 g protein.

DILLED VEGGIE DIP

EASY RECIPE:

1¼ cups plain fat-free yogurt

1 medium cucumber, peeled, seeded and chopped

3⁄4 cup light dairy sour cream

1 tbsp. snipped fresh dillweed or fresh mint

3 cloves garlic, minced

Salt and pepper

Assorted raw and/or chilled cooked vegetables

EASY STEPS:

In a food processor or blender container combine yogurt, cucumber, sour cream, dillweed or mint and garlic. Cover and process or blend until almost smooth. Season to taste with salt and pepper. Cover and chill for at least 2 hours. Serve with assorted vegetables. Makes 8 servings.

Nutrition facts per serving: 116 calories (14% from fat), 2 g total fat (1 g saturated fat), 4 mg cholesterol, 82 mg sodium, 20 g carbohydrate, 4 g dietary fiber, 7 g protein.

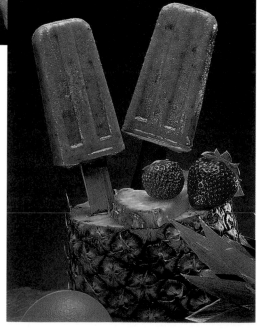

CRISP GARLIC POTATO SKINS

EASY RECIPE:

2 large baking potatoes

2 tsp. olive or cooking oil

2 medium tomatoes, seeded and chopped

1/4 tsp. dried basil, crushed

1/8 tsp. garlic powder

2 tsp. finely shredded or grated Parmesan cheese

Sliced green onion tops (optional)

EASY STEPS:

Several hours before serving prick the potatoes with a fork. Bake in a 425° oven for 40 to 50 minutes or until tender. Cool. Wrap and store in the refrigerator.

At serving time cut the baked potatoes into quarters. Scoop out the insides (reserve for another use), leaving 1/2-inch-thick shells.

Lightly brush both sides of potato quarters with olive oil. Place potato quarters, cut side up, on a large baking sheet. Bake in a 425° oven about 15 minutes or until crisp.

Meanwhile, in a small bowl combine chopped tomatoes, basil and garlic powder. Spoon some of the tomato mixture into each potato shell. Sprinkle with Parmesan cheese.

Bake for 2 to 3 minutes more or until heated through. Garnish potato skins with sliced green onion tops, if desired.

Makes 4 servings.

Nutrition facts per serving: 150 calories (17% from fat), 3 g total fat (1 g saturated fat), 1 mg cholesterol, 33 mg sodium, 29 g carbohydrate, 3 g dietary fiber, 3 g protein.

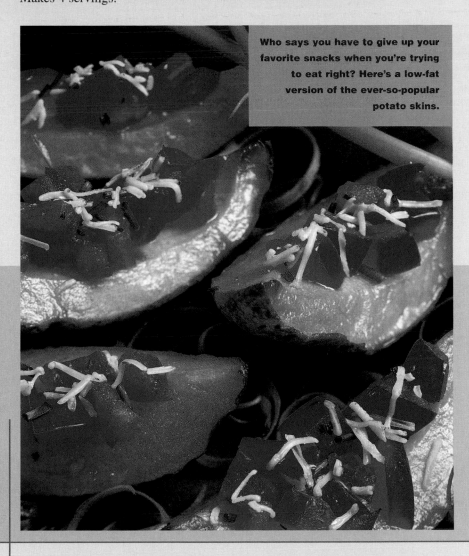

Who says you have to give up your favorite snacks when you're trying to eat right? Here's a low-fat version of the ever-so-popular potato skins.

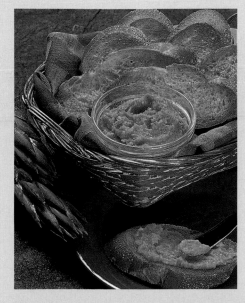

GARLIC ROASTED PURÉE

Garlic is a remarkable bulb. Use this roasted purée on bread, baked potatoes or grilled chicken.

EASY RECIPE:

4 heads garlic

1 tbsp. olive oil

1 tbsp. fresh lemon juice

1/4 tsp. salt

1/4 tsp. pepper

EASY STEPS:

Preheat oven to 350°F. Slice the bottom off heads of garlic to loosen cloves. Leave skins intact.

Place in shallow baking dish. Drizzle with olive oil. Bake for 20 minutes; cool. Press garlic from skins and place in food processor. Add lemon juice, salt and pepper. Process until smooth. Spread this mild purée on toasted French bread, baked potatoes or grilled chicken. Makes 4 servings.

Nutrition facts per serving: 82 calories (16% from fat), 3 g total fat (1g saturated fat), 0 mg cholesterol, 149 mg sodium, 12 g carbohydrate, 0 g dietary fiber, 1g protein.

savor these
smart suppers

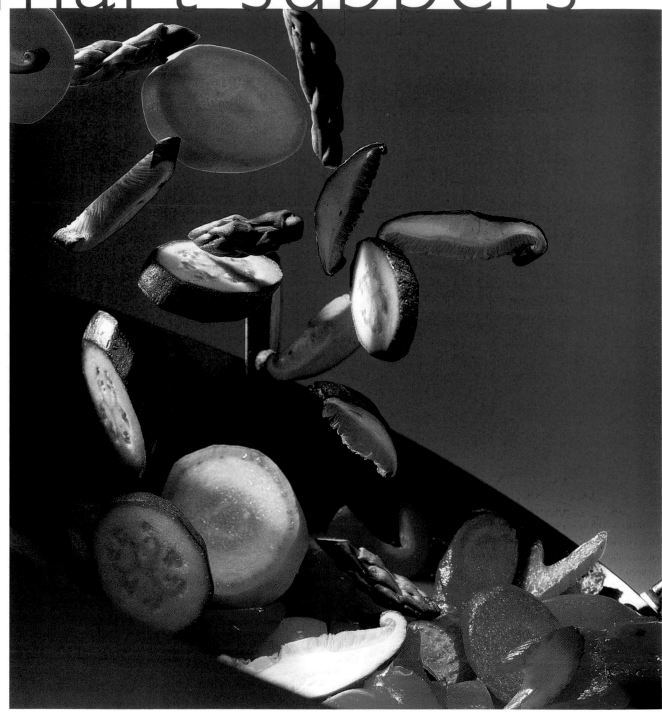

Become an expert at serving lively, nourishing meals.
Each of these standouts has fewer than 30 percent of its calories from fat
and is one full serving of a fruit or vegetable.

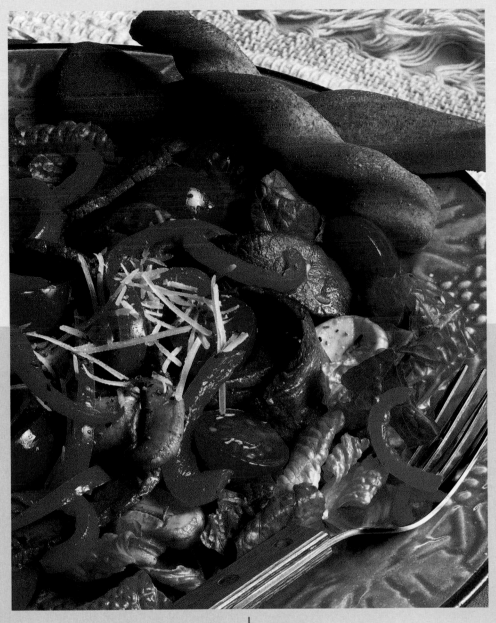

Dash freshly ground black
pepper (optional)

Shredded Parmesan cheese (optional)

EASY STEPS:

Cut steak crosswise into 1-inch-
wide strips; cut each strip in half
crosswise. Place the romaine in a
large bowl. Spray an unheated,
heavy, 12-inch nonstick skillet with
nonstick coating. Preheat over
medium heat. Add mushrooms,
sweet pepper and garlic to skillet;
stir-fry for 2 to 3 minutes or until
vegetables are crisp-tender. Remove
vegetables; remove skillet from
heat. Sprinkle vegetables with 1
teaspoon of the Italian seasoning,
stirring to combine; set aside.

In the same skillet, heat oil over
medium-high heat. Stir-fry beef
strips, half at a time, in oil for 1 to
1½ minutes. (Do not overcook.)
Remove meat; sprinkle with the salt
and set aside. Remove skillet from
heat; add tomatoes, vinegar and the
remaining Italian seasoning, stirring
to combine. Return beef and
vegetables to skillet; stir to combine.

Spoon beef mixture and pan juices
over romaine. Toss and serve
immediately. Sprinkle each serving
with freshly ground black pepper
and Parmesan cheese, if desired.
Makes 4 servings.

Nutrition facts per serving: 181 calories
(29% from fat), 6 g total fat (2 g saturated fat),
54 mg cholesterol, 341 mg sodium, 10 g
carbohydrate, 3 g dietary fiber, 23 g protein.

To make slicing the meat easier, place it in the freezer about 20 minutes or until partially frozen. Then, cut into strips.

QUICK ITALIAN-STYLE BEEF SALAD

EASY RECIPE:

12 oz. beef round tip steak, cut 1/8-to 1/4-inch thick

6 cups torn romaine

1½ cups sliced fresh mushrooms

1 medium green or yellow sweet pepper, cut into thin strips

2 cloves garlic, minced

1¼ tsp. dried Italian seasoning, crushed

1 tsp. olive oil

1/2 tsp. salt

1½ cups halved cherry tomato

2 tbsp. red wine vinegar

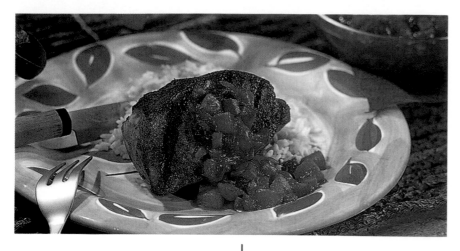

SPICY PORK CHOPS WITH NECTARINE MANGO SALSA

Spice-rubbed pork chops paired with a colorful fruit salsa make for a spicy-sweet dish. If you like your food hot, use the 2 tablespoons chili powder.

EASY RECIPE:

1 to 2 tbsp. chili powder

1/2 tsp. fajita seasoning

1/2 tsp. salt

1/2 tsp. pepper

4 (6-oz.) boneless pork chops, 1 to 1¼ inches thick

1 nectarine, pitted and coarsely chopped

1 mango, peeled, pitted and coarsely chopped

1/3 cup cherry or apricot preserves

EASY STEPS:

Preheat a covered grill to medium-hot. Combine chili powder, fajita seasoning, salt and pepper. Rub on all sides of chops.

Prepare grill for indirect cooking. Place chops on grill rack directly over medium heat. Cover and cook for 25 to 30 minutes, turning once or until juices run clear (160°F).

Meanwhile, combine nectarine, mango and preserves. Serve over pork chops.
Makes 4 servings.

Nutrition facts per serving: 382 calories, 10 g fat (4 sat. fat), 92 mg cholesterol, 414 mg sodium, 32 g carbohydrate, 2.5 g fiber, 38 g. protein.

PESTO SHRIMP AND SUMMER SQUASH

EASY RECIPE:

12 to 16 oz. peeled and deveined extra large raw shrimp

1 medium yellow summer squash, sliced

1 medium zucchini, sliced

1/3 cup purchased pesto

6 ounces dried angel hair pasta

EASY STEPS:

Preheat grill to medium. Place shrimp, summer squash and zucchini in center of an 18x36-inch piece of heavy-duty foil. Spoon pesto evenly over all. Bring edges of foil together and seal.

Grill foil packet for 8 to 10 minutes or until heated through and squash is just tender.

Meanwhile, cook pasta according to package directions. Drain and keep warm. Toss hot cooked pasta with shrimp and squash mixture.

If desired, add oiled or buttered French bread slices to the grill. Grill for about 1 minute per side. Makes 6 servings.

Nutrition facts per serving: 346 calories, protein 22 g, 12 g fat, 2 g saturated fat, 108 mg cholesterol, 252 mg sodium, 37 g carbohydrates, 2 g fiber.

This zesty pasta topper cooks on the grill in a foil packet. Brush slices of French bread with olive oil and grill until toasty. Serve the bread alongside this colorful pasta entrée.

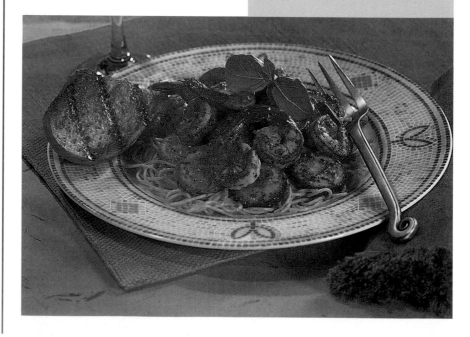

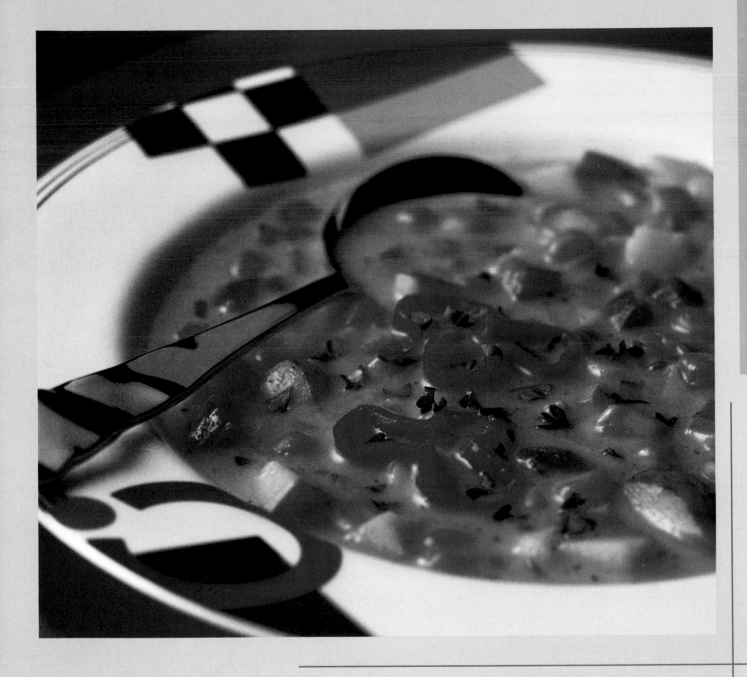

CORN CHOWDER

A fresh variation on a hearty comfort food, this chowder is filling, yet low in calories and fat.

EASY RECIPE:

2 pounds white potatoes, diced

1 bay leaf

3 tbsp. margarine or butter

3 medium onions, chopped

4 celery ribs, chopped

1 medium green pepper, chopped

2 tsp. cumin seeds

3 tbsp. flour

1/2 tsp. each dried sage, crushed, and white pepper

2 cups low-fat (1%) milk

1⅔ cups cooked fresh or frozen whole kernel corn

EASY STEPS:

In a large covered saucepan combine potatoes, bay leaf and 4 cups water; bring to a boil. Cook, covered, 15 minutes or just until potatoes are tender. Discard bay leaf. Drain potatoes, reserving liquid. Set aside. In same saucepan melt margarine. Add next 4 ingredients; cook until onions are tender. Stir in flour, sage and white pepper. Stir in enough reserved potato liquid to make a paste. Stir in remaining potato liquid and potatoes. **Heat through.** Stir in milk and corn; heat through. Top with snipped parsley and red pepper slices, if desired. Makes 14 servings.

Nutrition facts per serving: **150 calories** (19% from fat), 3 g total fat, 1 mg cholesterol, 80 mg sodium, 28 g carbohydrate, 2 g dietary fiber, 4 g protein.

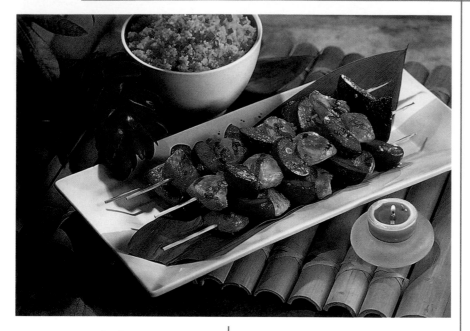

PLUM SAUCED CHICKEN KABOBS

If you prefer these chicken and plum skewers with a sweet-tart taste, use orange marmalade instead of plum jam in the brushing sauce.

EASY RECIPE:

1 lb. skinless, boneless chicken breast halves, cut in 1-inch pieces

4 quartered plums

1/2 cup plum jam

2 thinly sliced green onions

1½ tsp. prepared horseradish

EASY STEPS:

Preheat grill to medium. Alternately thread chicken and plums on four 12- to 15-inch skewers.

Combine plum jam, green onion and horseradish.

Grill kabobs 10 to 12 minutes or until chicken is tender and no longer pink, turning once. Brush with half of the plum jam mixture during the last 5 minutes of grilling time.

Brush kabobs with remaining jam mixture. Serve over couscous tossed with sliced green onion, if desired. Makes 4 servings.

Nutrition facts per serving: 234 calories, 2 g fat (0.5 sat. fat), 43 mg cholesterol, 58 mg sodium, 37 g carbohydrates, 2 g fiber, 18 g protein.

SNAPPER WITH WARM PINEAPPLE SALSA

A fresh jalapeño pepper gives this colorful salsa a pleasant kick. Another time, try the versatile salsa with a different variety of fish or grilled chicken or pork chops.

EASY RECIPE:

2½ cups bite-sized pieces fresh pineapple

1/2 cup chopped red bell pepper

1 jalapeño pepper, finely chopped*

2 tbsp. thawed frozen orange juice concentrate

4 (5-to 6-oz.) red snapper fillets with skin (1/2 to 3/4 inch thick)

1 tbsp. chopped fresh cilantro

EASY STEPS:

Preheat grill to medium. Spray grill rack with nonstick cooking spray. Brush the fish fillets with 2 tsp. of the orange juice concentrate and sprinkle with pepper. Fold a 36x18-inch piece of heavy foil in half crosswise. Place pineapple, red pepper and jalapeño pepper in center and toss with remaining orange juice concentrate. Bring up edges and seal.

Place the pineapple packet on the grill and cook for 10 minutes or until pineapple is hot.

Grill fish alongside the foil packet. Grill for 5 minutes per half inch of thickness, turning once or until fish flakes with a fork.

Carefully open foil packet and sprinkle pineapple with cilantro. Serve with fish.
Makes 4 servings.

*Use caution when handling hot peppers. Wear disposable gloves or wash hands thoroughly with hot soapy water.

NOTE: If your snapper does not have skin on one side, grill on a lightly greased grill topper designed for fish.

Nutrition facts per serving: 151 calories, 2 g fat (0.3 sat. fat), 26 mg cholesterol, 67 mg sodium, 18 g carbohydrates, 2 g fiber, 16 g protein.

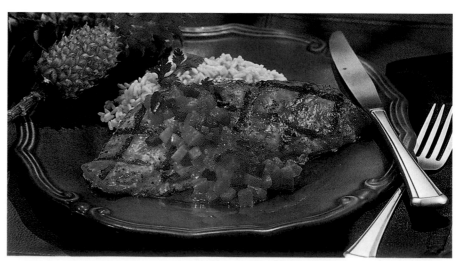

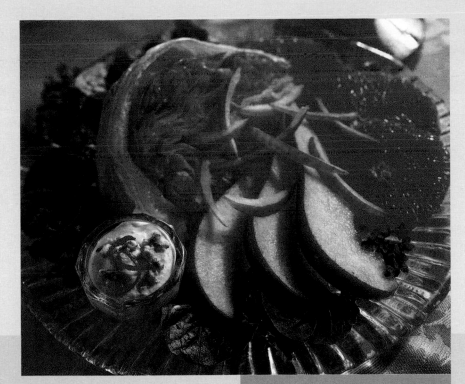

BELL PEPPER STUFFED WITH TURKEY

A filling of ground turkey, rice, raisins and tomato sauce gives a Mediterranean flair to these stuffed peppers.

EASY RECIPE:

4 large red or green bell peppers

1 medium chopped onion

2 cloves garlic, minced

1½ tbsp. olive oil

1 lb. ground turkey

1½ cups cooked rice

1/4 cup raisins

1 (15-oz.) can tomato sauce

1 tbsp. chopped parsley

Salt and pepper

EASY STEPS:

Preheat oven to 350°F. Cut stem end from peppers. Remove seeds. Cook covered in boiling water for 1 minute. Drain. In skillet, cook onions and garlic in olive oil until soft. Add turkey and cook until no longer pink. Drain fat. In bowl, combine turkey, rice, raisins, half of the tomato sauce and parsley. Season to taste with salt and pepper. Stuff the peppers and place upright in a 2-quart casserole. Spoon remaining tomato sauce on the peppers. Cover and cook for 30 minutes.

Makes 4 servings.

Nutrition facts per serving: 352 calories (22% from fat), 9 g total fat, 67 mg cholesterol, 410 mg sodium, 38 g carbohydrate, 4 g dietary fiber, 31 g protein.

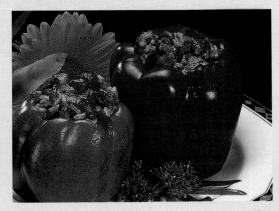

SUNSATIONAL CITRUS SALAD

EASY RECIPE:

Bleu Cheese Dressing

3/4 cup low-fat cottage cheese

3 tbsp. nonfat dry milk powder

2 tbsp. cold water

2 tbsp. crumbled bleu cheese

4 tsp. fresh lemon juice

1/4 tsp. onion powder

Dash garlic powder

Salad

1 head iceberg lettuce

Mixed salad greens (optional)

2 or 3 large oranges

2 medium pears

1 medium sweet red onion, cut into thin strips

Orange peel strips (optional)

EASY STEPS:

To make the dressing: In a food processor bowl combine the cottage cheese, nonfat dry milk powder, water, bleu cheese, lemon juice, onion powder and garlic powder. Cover and process with a stop-and-

Using low-fat cottage cheese and nonfat dry milk powder keeps the bleu cheese dressing low in fat, and also gives it a creamy, rich body.

go motion until the mixture is almost smooth, scraping sides of bowl frequently. Cover and chill at least 2 hours.

To make the salad: Core, rinse and thoroughly drain lettuce; refrigerate in an airtight container. To serve, line 4 salad plates with some of the outer iceberg lettuce leaves or mixed greens, if desired. Cut the head of iceberg lettuce into wedges. Peel oranges and slice cartwheel style. Core and cut pears into thin wedges. Arrange lettuce wedges, fruit and onion on salad plates. Serve each salad with some of the dressing. Garnish with orange peel strips, if desired. Pass remaining dressing. Makes 4 servings.

Nutrition facts per serving: 171 calories (12% from fat), 2 g total fat (1 g saturated fat), 6 mg cholesterol, 262 mg sodium, 30 g carbohydrate, 6 g dietary fiber, 10 g protein.

sweet
splurges

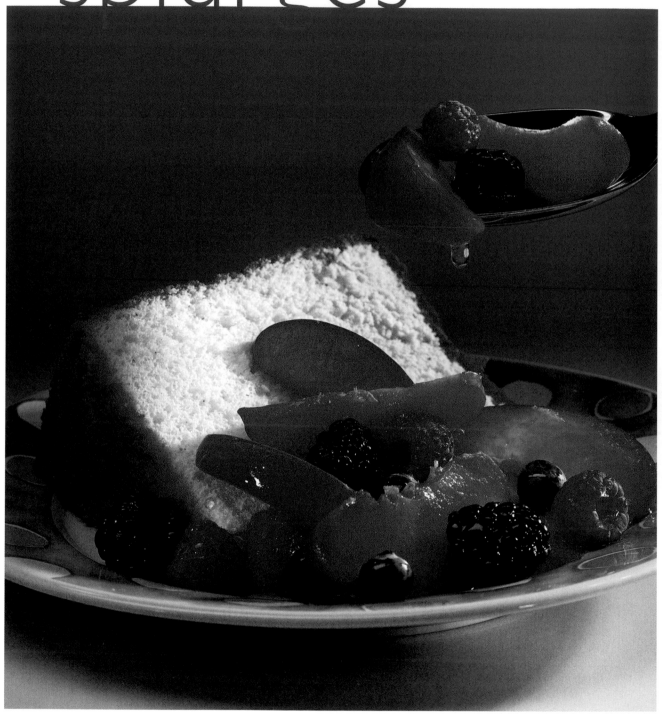

Go ahead and splurge! Here you'll find the pick of the crop of
after-dinner delectables. Each dessert is low in fat and calories,
yet high in flavor and freshness.

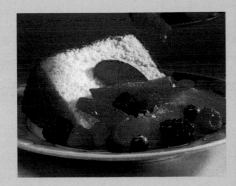

HEAVENLY SUMMER CAKE

Fresh fruit and angel cake team up for a glamorous, luscious dessert.

EASY RECIPE:

1 purchased angel food cake (about 1 pound), cut into 1/2-inch-thick slices with crust removed

1/3 cup fresh orange juice or white grape juice

1/4 cup sugar

4 cups fresh raspberries

2 cups peeled and chopped fresh peaches

EASY STEPS:

Arrange about three-fourths of the cake slices on the bottom and sides of an 8-cup soufflé dish, overlapping or cutting pieces to fit; set aside. In a small saucepan stir together orange juice and sugar; heat just until sugar dissolves. Remove from heat. Stir in the raspberries and peaches. Pour fruit mixture into cake-lined soufflé dish. Cover with remaining cake slices. Cover with waxed paper. Place a heavy plate on top of waxed paper. Weigh the plate down with a heavy object, such as a can of fruit or a pan. Chill overnight. To serve remove the weight, plate and paper. Gently loosen edges of pudding with a thin-bladed knife. Invert onto a serving plate.
Makes 10 servings.

Nutrition facts per serving: 149 calories (3% from fat), 1 g total fat (0 g saturated fat), 0 mg cholesterol, 254 mg sodium, 35 g carbohydrate, 3 g dietary fiber, 3 g protein.

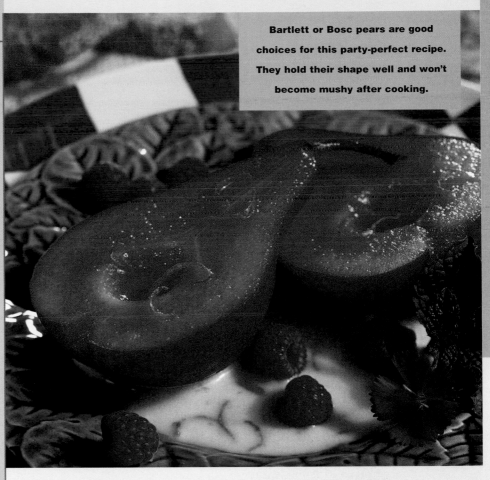

Bartlett or Bosc pears are good choices for this party-perfect recipe. They hold their shape well and won't become mushy after cooking.

BAKED PEARS WITH LEMON SAUCE

EASY RECIPE:

Lemon Sauce

3/4 cup skim milk

2 tsp. cornstarch

3 inches stick cinnamon

1 tbsp. honey

1 tsp. grated lemon peel

Honey Pears

4 medium pears, peeled

3 tbsp. water

1 tbsp. honey

2 whole cloves

Fresh raspberries (optional)

Lemon peel strips (optional)

EASY STEPS:

To make the sauce: In a small saucepan stir together 1/4 cup of the milk and the cornstarch. Stir in the remaining 1/2 cup of milk and stick cinnamon. Cook over medium heat, stirring constantly, for 6 to 8 minutes or until the mixture is thickened and bubbly. Reduce heat and stir in honey and lemon peel. Remove from heat and cool to room temperature. Cover and chill about 3 hours or until thoroughly chilled. Discard stick cinnamon.

To prepare the pears: Cut pears in half lengthwise and remove cores. Arrange pears, cut side up, in a 3-quart rectangular baking dish. In a small bowl combine water, honey and cloves; pour over pears. Bake, covered, in a 350° oven for 25 to 30 minutes or until the pears are tender. Discard the cloves. Serve the warm pears with the chilled lemon sauce. Garnish each serving with raspberries and lemon peel strips, if desired.
Makes 4 servings.

Nutrition facts per serving: 152 calories (4% from fat), 1 g total fat (0 g saturated fat), 1 mg cholesterol, 25 mg sodium, 37 g carbohydrate, 5 g dietary fiber, 2 g protein.

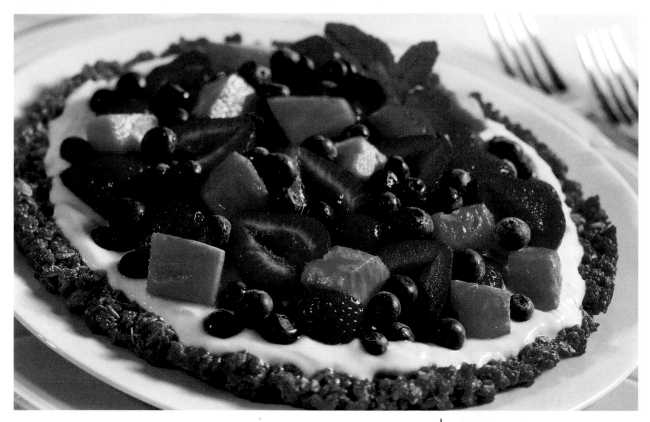

(cover recipe)

FRUIT AND CRÈME TART

This light, airy dessert, overflowing with fresh fruit, makes a colorful climax to any great meal.

EASY RECIPE:

1/4 cup water

1 egg white

2½ cups low-fat granola without raisins

1 tsp. butter or margarine

2 cartons (8 oz. each) low-fat vanilla, lemon or pineapple yogurt

2 cups fresh strawberries, halved

1 cup fresh blueberries

1 cup fresh pineapple cubes

Fresh mint (optional)

EASY STEPS:

Preheat oven to 350⁰F. To make granola crust, in medium bowl beat together water and egg white; stir in granola. Continue stirring until all liquid is absorbed.

Coat the bottom of a 9- or 10-inch tart pan* with removable sides with butter or margarine. Pat granola mixture evenly into bottom of pan.
Bake for 12 minutes.
Cool completely.

Just before serving spoon yogurt over granola crust. Gently top with strawberries, blueberries and pineapple. Garnish with fresh mint, if desired.
Makes 6 to 8 servings.

*Or use a 10-inch oven-safe platter.

Nutrition facts per serving: 203 cal. 3 g fat (1 sat. fat), 4 mg cholesterol, 126 mg sodium, 39 g carbohydrate, 4 g fiber, 6 g protein.

Be imaginative! Try Grand Marnier or any other favorite liqueur and any kind of fruit that you like.

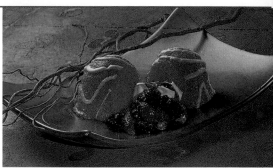

LEMON CAKE WITH FRUIT COMPOTE

EASY RECIPE:

1/2 (24-oz.) bakery lemon cream cake

5 cups berries (blackberries, strawberries, blueberries or raspberries)

1/3 cup brandy, Grand Marnier or liqueur

1/2 (8-oz.) carton frozen fat-free whipped topping, thawed

EASY STEPS:

Cut cake into 12 pieces. To make compote, simmer berries in brandy until berries are soft. Cool.

Spoon compote over each piece of cake. Garnish with whipped topping.
Makes 8 servings.

Nutrition facts per serving: 227 calories, 7 g fat (1.5 saturated fat), 26 mg cholesterol, 137 mg sodium, 33 g carbohydrate, 3 g dietary fiber, 2 g protein.

STARS-N-STRIPES FRUIT GRILL

Star fruit, also known as carambola, is fun in star shapes as garnish. Serve this colorful fruit grill with grilled chicken, pork or beef dishes.

EASY RECIPE:

2 carambola (star fruit), sliced 1/2-inch thick

1 pineapple, peeled, cored and sliced into 1-inch rings

4 peaches or nectarines, pitted and halved

2 tbsp. brown sugar

1 tbsp. orange juice

1 cup raspberries or blueberries

EASY STEPS:

Place carambola, pineapple and peaches directly on a lightly oiled, heated grill. Cook 3 to 4 minutes, watching carefully to avoid burning. Turn and grill until golden brown. Mix together brown sugar and orange juice. Add raspberries. Place grilled fruit on 4 dessert plates. Top each with some of raspberry mixture.
Makes 4 servings.

Nutrition facts per serving: **141 calories** (6% from fat), 1 g total fat, 0 mg cholesterol, 6 mg sodium, 36 g carbohydrate, 1 g dietary fiber, 2 g protein.

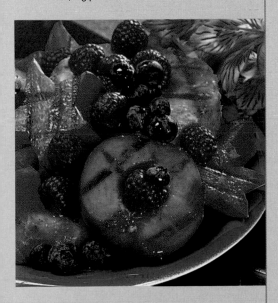

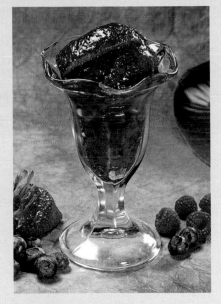

BERRY SORBET

To add a touch of elegance to any meal, serve scoops of this refreshing ice in crystal dessert dishes. Top each serving with a few berries.

EASY RECIPE:

3/4 cup unsweetened apple juice or fresh orange juice

3 tbsp. sugar

PEACHES FRANÇAIS

Drizzle a citrus-scented wine syrup over fresh peach slices for a luscious fat-free, low-calorie dessert.

EASY RECIPE:

1/2 vanilla bean (or 1 tsp. pure vanilla extract)

1½ cups red wine

1/2 lemon, sliced

1/2 orange, sliced

1/4 cup honey

6 ripe peaches, peeled and sliced

6 sprigs of mint

EASY STEPS:

With a sharp knife, slice vanilla bean in half lengthwise. Scrape small, sticky seeds from the pod.

Combine wine, lemon, orange, honey and vanilla seeds (or extract) in a stainless steel saucepan.

3 cups fresh blueberries, raspberries or strawberries

1 tsp. fresh lime juice

EASY STEPS:

In a small saucepan combine juice and sugar. Bring to a boil and cook for 1 minute. Remove from heat and cool to room temperature.

In a blender container combine the berries and 1/4 cup of the juice mixture. Cover and blend until smooth. In a large mixing bowl, stir together the puréed berries, the remaining 1/2 cup of the juice mixture and lime juice until combined. Pour mixture into freezer can of a hand-turned or electric freezer. Freeze according to manufacturer's directions.
Makes 6 servings.

Nutrition facts per serving: **47 calories** (0% from fat), 0 g total fat (0 g saturated fat), 0 mg cholesterol, 1 mg sodium, 11 g carbohydrate, 1 g dietary fiber, 1 g protein.

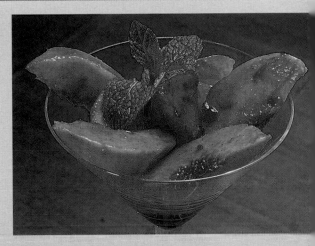

Bring mixture to a boil over medium-high heat for 3 minutes. Remove from heat and cool completely. Divide peaches between 6 large martini or wine glasses. Strain wine syrup over the peaches. Garnish with mint.
Makes 6 servings.

Nutrition facts per serving: **110 calories** (0% from fat), 0 g total fat (less than 20 g saturated fat), 0 mg cholesterol, 5 mg sodium, 26 g carbohydrate, 3 g dietary fiber, 1 g protein.

glossary

A

Alpha and beta carotene – Precursors to vitamin A.

Anthocyanins – Powerful antioxidants that inhibit blood clot formation.

Antioxidant – A compound that protects against oxidation damage.

Absorption – The saturation of nutrients into intestinal cells.

B

Balanced diet – The proportionate consumption of foods which is necessary for proper growth and good health.

Beta carotene – An orange pigment associated with vitamin A, found in certain plants.

Beta cryptoxanthin – A carotenoid believed to offer cancer-fighting properties.

Boron – A mineral important for calcium absorption.

C

Carotenoids – Pigments commonly found in plants and animals, usually having biological activity in the body (Alpha, Beta).

Chronic disease – Degenerative diseases characterized by deterioration of body organs, i.e., cancer, heart, diabetes.

Cruciferous – Vegetables from the cabbage family, i.e., Bok Choy, broccoli, Brussels sprouts, cabbage, cauliflower, Chinese cabbage, collard greens, kale, kohlrabi, radishes, rutabaga, Swiss chard and turnips.

D

Deficiency – Below standard nutrient levels over a period of time.

Dermatitis – A skin condition.

E

Edema – A result of deficiency in protein or thiamin, wherein a swelling of tissue caused by body fluid retention occurs.

Ellagic acid – A natural substance found in some berries that preliminary research suggests may help prevent certain types of cancer.

Endothelium – A thin layer of flattened cells that line internal body cavities.

F

FDA – The Food & Drug Administration.

Fiber – Found in grain products and fruit and vegetables, such as apples, broccoli, grapefruit, mango, papaya and peas. May aid in prevention of some types of cancers.

Fitness – The ability to perform physical activity, challenging the body to withstand stress or endurance.

Flavonoid – A phytochemical that acts as an antioxidant reducing the risk of cancer.

Folate – A B vitamin, also known as folic acid, especially necessary for fetal development.

Fortified – Food that has been altered to balance the nutrient level.

G

Gram (g) – A measurement of .04 ounce.

I

Indoles – A phytochemical that triggers an enzyme to inhibit estrogen action, a function that may reduce the risk of breast cancer.

Isothiocyanate – A micronutrient that can block carcinogenic activity in the body.

K

Kilogram (kg) – A measurement of 1,000 grams.

L

Legumes – Of the bean and pea family, rich in protein.

Limonene – A phytochemical found in citrus that triggers enzyme production to facilitate carcinogen excretion.

Lycopene
Lycopene – A phytochemical found in red pigmented fruits and vegetables, may aid in the prevention of certain types of cancer.

Lutein – A phytochemical found in yellow pigmented fruits and vegetables, may promote good vision.

M

Microgram (mcg) – A measurement of 1/1000 of a milligram.

Milligram (mg) – A measurement of 1/1000 of a gram.

Mineral – Essential nutrients required in one's diet. Major minerals include calcium, chloride, magnesium, phosphorus, potassium, sodium and sulfur.

N

Nutrients – Sources of energy obtained from food. Regulate growth, maintenance and repair of tissue.

O

Organic – Produce grown without fertilizers, pesticides or chemicals.

Oxidation – A process in which a substance combines with oxygen.

P

Pectin – A soluble fiber that is effective in lowering cholesterol levels.

Phenol – A type of antioxidant that helps to fight against chronic diseases.

Phytochemicals – Non-nutrient plant chemicals that have a biological effect in the body.

Potassium – A principal component critical to maintain fluid balance, nerve transmission and muscle contractions.

Q

Quercitin – A member of the bioflavonoid family, a group of coloring pigments that provide plants antioxidant protection against environmental stress.

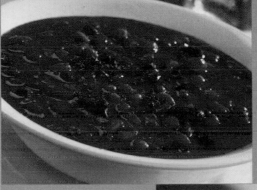

R

RDA – Recommended Dietary Allowances.

Resveratrol – A compound, found largely in the skins of red grapes. Preliminary studies indicate beneficial cardiovascular and cancer-related effects.

S

Scurvy – An extreme deficiency of vitamin C.

Sulforaphane – A micronutrient that breaks down excretion of carcinogens in the liver.

Supplements – Pills, liquids or powders that contain purified nutrients.

T

Toxins – Chemicals in certain food products that may cause ill effects on the human body.

U

USDA – The United States Department of Agriculture.

V

Vegetarians – People who omit meat, seafood and other animal by-products from their diets.

Vitamin – Organic, essential nutrients required in small amounts by the body for health.

Z

Zeaxanthin – A phytochemical found in yellow pigmented fruits and vegetables. May promote good vision.

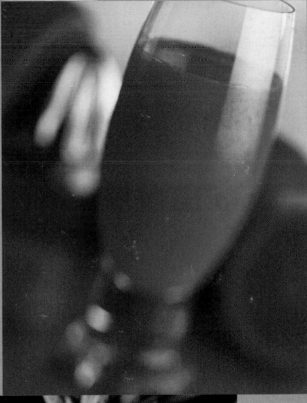

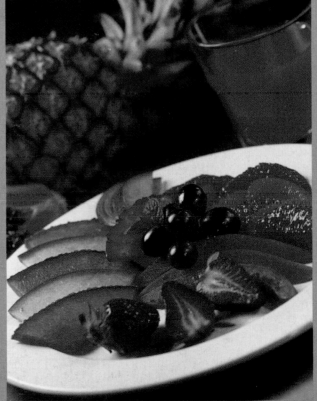

index

INDEX

93

There is a tremendous amount of literature to read on well-being.

Several web sites are available to aide you in your journey toward healthy living. Log on to these recommended sites:

www.nih.gov - National Institutes of Health - provides information about rare diseases, drugs and clinical trials.

www.mayoclinic.com - Mayo Clinic - offers answers to questions about disease management, drugs, first aid and weight loss, exercise tips and smoking cessation hints.

www.nlm.nih.gov - National Library of Medicine - condenses research studies by reviewing citations from thousands of medical journals.

www.americanheart.org - American Heart Association - instructs about heart conditions and stroke symptoms; get diet and exercise plans for disease prevention.

www.webmd.com - WebMD - a doctor's advice is just a keystroke away.

www.aboutproduce.com - About Produce - features top produce items; nutrition facts, seasonality, information and recipes.

www.dole5aday.com - Dole - offers teachers and families super tips and activities to make produce fun.

www.pma.com - Produce Marketing Association - outlines events and activities for professionals in the produce industry.

www.5aday.com - Produce for Better Health® Foundation - navigates through the 5 A Day mission, kids activities, healthy recipes.